Protection and Prevention Approaches in Occupational Health and Safety

Edited by Hülya Gül

Published in London, United Kingdom

Protection and Prevention Approaches in Occupational Health and Safety
http://dx.doi.org/10.5772/intechopen.111124
Edited by Hülya Gül

Contributors
Ali Faghihi Zarandi, Amsalu Taye, Bekele Getenet Tiruneh, Dmitry Olegovich Lastkov, Ehsan Garosi, Fatemeh Sheikh, Inna Sergeevna Eromyants, Mahdi Jalali, Mahsa Goodarzi, Martin Popević, Mengistu Abebe Messelu, Mohammad Amin Rajizadeh, Mohammad Bagher Hasanvand, Mohsen Sadeghi-Yarandi, Oleg Viktorovich Partas, Olga Yurievna Nikolenko, Reza Pourbabaki, Temesgen Ayenew, Zabiholah Damiri, Zhaleh Sedghi Noushabadi

First published in London, United Kingdom, 2025 by IntechOpen
IntechOpen is the global imprint of INTECHOPEN LIMITED, registered in England and Wales, registration number: 11086078, 167-169 Great Portland Street, London, W1W 5PF, United Kingdom

For EU product safety concerns: IN TECH d.o.o., Prolaz Marije Krucifikse Kozulić 3, 51000 Rijeka, Croatia, info@intechopen.com or visit our website at intechopen.com.

British Library Cataloguing-in-Publication Data
A catalogue record for this book is available from the British Library

Protection and Prevention Approaches in Occupational Health and Safety
Edited by Hülya Gül
p. cm.

This title is part of the Public Health Book Series, Volume 3
Series Editor: José Antonio Mirón Canelo

Print ISBN 978-1-83634-116-1
Online ISBN 978-1-83634-115-4
eBook (PDF) ISBN 978-1-83634-117-8
ISSN 3049-8872

If disposing of this product, please recycle the paper responsibly.

IntechOpen Book Series
Public Health
Volume 3

Aims and Scope of the Series

Public health is what we as a society do collectively to contribute to and ensure the health and social conditions for the enjoyment of health as a resource for life. It can also be defined as science and research that promotes health, prevents disease, and improves populations' well-being and quality of life. Its objective is to know the risk factors that determine and condition the populations' health levels at present. At the end of the 20th century and the beginning of the 21st century, it is unjustifiable and regrettable that morbimortality according to age plays a leading role when the causes are mostly well known and therefore preventable, such as obesity, AIDS, cirrhosis, diabetes mellitus, addictions and cancer associated with the consumption of tobacco and alcohol, etc. In short, public health is science based on epidemiology and biostatistics, and currently, new technologies and artificial intelligence must be incorporated to identify patterns and trends in what we do collectively as a society to ensure living conditions and prevent risk factors that affect individual and population health. For all these reasons, it is essential to scientifically investigate and act on the determinants that impede the well-being and quality of life related to the health of people, patients, and populations in general, given that to control the determinants of diseases, it is important to control the environment and genetics. Consequently, the current fight for public health must prioritize the control of the environment, such as atmospheric and biological pollution and environmental and social biodiversity, promoting the sensitivity and training of society and its individuals by empowering them to make free and appropriate decisions about these aspects to lead healthy lifestyles based on motivation and responsibility in the face of the challenges they cope with from an individual point of view, such as dealing with the addictions that exist in today's complex world. Public health also requires an ethical vision and incorporates strategies to reduce social inequality.

Meet the Series Editor

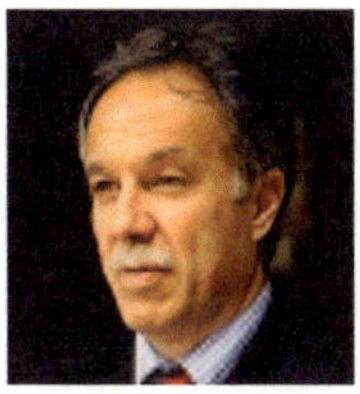

José Antonio Mirón Canelo is a physician, doctor, and professor of Preventive Medicine and Public Health at the Faculty of Medicine and Dentistry of the University of Salamanca with over 30 years of experience. He is the director of the USAL's Expert Degree in Health Management, currently in its 13th edition. Prof. Mirón Canelo directs a research group at the Research Institute of Biomedical Sciences (IBSAL) of the University of Salamanca focused on addressing the challenges and care needs of vulnerable people and patients such as the elderly with multiple pathologies and people with disabilities and dependence. As a teacher, he has been recognized for excellence in teaching three times in a period of five years.

Meet the Volume Editor

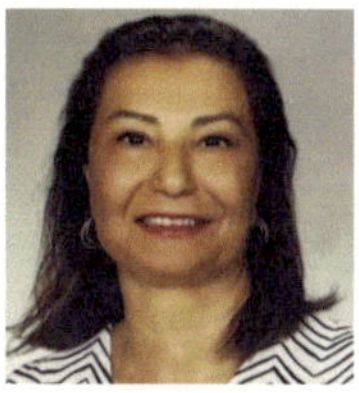

Prof. Dr. Hülya Gül earned two Doctorates of Medical Sciences from Istanbul University in Turkey. Her first one was from Istanbul University, Oncology Institute, Preventive Oncology Department. She completed her second doctorate in Istanbul Faculty of Medicine, Department of Public Health. Her research areas focus on public health, environmental health, occupational health, epidemiology, toxicology, and cancer. She has more than ten book chapters written nationally and internationally. She has more than fifty publications published in indexed journals and presented more than fifty papers at international congresses. She has taught and continues to teach undergraduate, doctoral and graduate students on these subjects at the medical school. She had been at Istanbul University, Faculty of Medicine, since enrolling there but left in 2024. That same year, she began working in the Department of Public Health within the Internal Medical Sciences division at Istanbul Aydın University.

Contents

Preface

Employees are exposed to various factors in the work environment, including physical, chemical, biological, psychological, and ergonomic influences, each in different forms and intensities. This book focuses on the hazards in the work environment, the risks they may create, and the precautions that can be taken to protect the health of employees and prevent deterioration. It has been prepared in light of current information, from a multidisciplinary perspective, and for application. The authors, occupational health and safety experts working in different countries, have addressed easily understandable, accessible solutions for dangerous and risky situations in line with their own experiences. The book consists of eight chapters with detailed topics to guide those interested in occupational health and safety. It covers important subjects like chemicals, disasters, stress, ergonomics, sleep apnea, noise, fibrogenic aerosols, and medical errors. Some negative aspects of these factors on employee health and methods to combat them are discussed.

Dr. Hülya Gül
Professor,
Internal Medical Sciences,
Istanbul Aydın University,
İstanbul, Türkiye

Chapter 1

Chemical Agents that Cause Occupational Diseases: Toxicity, Exposure Routes, and Health Effects

Reza Pourbabaki, Mohammad Amin Rajizadeh, Ali Faghihi Zarandi, Mohsen Sadeghi-Yarandi and Zabiholah Damiri

Abstract

Chemicals are widely used in daily activities and various industries. While they may seem harmless, they can actually have significant adverse health effects when they come into contact with the body or are used for prolonged periods of time. Occupational diseases (ODs) are illnesses contracted as a result of exposure to harmful factors in the workplace. The International Labour Organization (ILO) categorizes ODs into four principal groups: diseases caused by exposure to agents associated with work activities (e.g., chemical, physical, and biological agents); diseases targeting specific organ systems; occupational cancers; and other work-related diseases. Among these, chemical agents represent the most prevalent occupational hazards contributing to the development of ODs. This chapter will explore the toxicity of various chemicals, how they can enter the body, and the health effects they can cause. It will specifically focus on occupational diseases and cancers caused by chemical agents. Additionally, the chapter will discuss the importance of preventive measures in the workplace to reduce these risks. Understanding the mechanisms of toxicity and implementing effective preventive strategies are essential to decreasing the incidence of chemical-related occupational diseases.

Keywords: occupational diseases, chemical agents, toxicity, exposure routes, preventive measures

1. Introduction

Chemicals play a crucial role in our daily lives and various industries [1]. They are essential for producing a wide range of products, including pharmaceuticals, paints, detergents, and plastics. However, it is important to note that even seemingly harmless chemicals can cause injury upon contact. In some cases, adverse health effects may manifest only after prolonged exposure and a certain period [2, 3].

An occupational disease (OD) is defined as a disease contracted due to exposure to factors related to work activity [4, 5]. To diagnose OD, it is necessary to establish a causal relationship between exposure in a specific work environment or activity and the onset of a specific disease. Additionally, the disease must occur with a higher frequency among exposed individuals compared to the average morbidity rate in the general population. The International Labour Organization (ILO) categorizes ODs into four main groups: those caused by exposure to agents arising from work activities (such as physical, chemical, and biological agents), those affecting specific organ systems, occupational cancers, and other diseases [6].

Chemical agents are responsible for 41% of occupational diseases caused by exposure to work-related agents, making them the most prevalent occupational hazard leading to disease. Moreover, chemical agents play a significant role in occupational diseases affecting specific organ systems, particularly respiratory and skin diseases, as well as occupational cancers [6–8].

This entry focuses on the toxicity of chemicals and their various health effects, including ODs and cancer. It discusses routes of exposure and preventive measures in the workplace.

2. Toxicity of chemical agents

Toxicology is the study of how poisons affect the body. Toxicity refers to a chemical's ability to cause injury or disease in a living organism due to its interaction with living tissue [9]. It's important to recognize that all substances, including chemicals, have the potential to be poisonous. However, if exposure to chemicals is kept below tolerable limits, they can be used safely [10]. Several factors influence the toxicity and health effects of a chemical. These factors include the physical state of the chemical, its size or aerodynamic diameter, the duration and concentration of exposure, the presence of other chemicals, and the route of absorption. Personal factors also play a role in determining a worker's susceptibility to the adverse effects of a chemical. These factors include genetics, gender, age, hypersensitivity, personal habits and hygiene, overall health status, and whether the individual is pregnant or lactating [11, 12].

3. Hazard classification of chemicals

A hazard refers to anything that could potentially cause bodily harm. This includes physical, chemical, mechanical, biological, electrical, and ergonomic hazards. The Globally Harmonized System (GHS) categorizes hazardous chemicals in the workplace into three types: health hazards, physical hazards, and environmental hazards (**Table 1**) [13, 14].

4. Routes of exposure

Chemicals can enter the human body through inhalation, ingestion, or contact with the skin. Inhalation and dermal exposure are the primary ways that people are exposed to hazardous substances in the workplace [15].

Hazard types	Hazard categories
Health hazard	Skin corrosion/irritation; skin sensitizer (including dermal exposure); serious eye irritation/eye damage; acute toxicity (oral and inhalation); respiratory sensitizer; carcinogenicity; mutagenicity; toxicity to reproduction; aspiration hazard; specific target organ toxicity (following single exposure); specific target organ toxicity (following repeated exposure).
Physical hazard	Explosives; flammable aerosols; flammable liquids; flammable gases; flammable solids; gases under pressure; oxidizing gases; pyrophoric liquids; pyrophoric solids; self-heating substances; self-reactive substances; substances which, on contact with water, emit flammable gases; oxidizing solids; oxidizing liquids; corrosive to metals organic peroxides
Environmental hazard	Chronic and acute hazards to the aquatic environment

Table 1.
Globally Harmonized System hazard classes.

Inhaling airborne chemical agents, such as gases, vapors, and particulate matter (dust, aerosols, fumes, smoke, and mists), can lead to rapid absorption into the lungs and subsequent circulation throughout the body, affecting various organs [16].

The rate of absorption through the skin is typically slower compared to inhalation or ingestion. However, if there is a cut or wound on the skin, dermal absorption can occur rapidly. Numerous chemical compounds, particularly lipophilic substances, can permeate intact skin. Moreover, dermal exposure to hazardous chemical agents may result in the development of occupational skin diseases [17, 18].

Chemicals can be absorbed through the skin without the worker even noticing. Certain chemicals commonly used in the workplace, like pesticides and organic solvents, have the potential to cause harm throughout the body if they penetrate the skin and enter the bloodstream. Workers sometimes have misconceptions about how chemicals enter their bodies, based on the chemicals' properties. For example, some workers mistakenly believe that if a pesticide has a strong smell, the main route of entry is through inhalation. They think that wearing a mask would protect them from absorption. However, pesticides that are fat-soluble are primarily absorbed through the skin and mucous membranes. In these cases, workers must wear protective clothing for their skin, including gloves and eye protection [19].

Toxic chemical compounds can enter the bloodstream through the digestive system. Workers in the workplace can unknowingly ingest these chemicals. For example, some workers may eat or drink without realizing that their hands are contaminated. Another common example is when workers handle cigarettes with contaminated hands while smoking, resulting in unintentional ingestion of the chemicals [20].

5. Health effects

Toxic chemicals can lead to health effects that are either local or systemic. Local effects occur at the specific area of contact with the body, like irritating the skin or eyes. On the other hand, systemic effects occur at a different location in the body from where the chemicals initially entered, such as damaging the liver or kidneys. Health effects can occur either immediately or over time. Immediate effects, known as acute effects, result from short-term, high-level exposure. On the other hand, chronic effects are health issues that develop after repeated exposure to chemicals. Exposure to chemicals can result in either reversible or irreversible health effects. Reversible effects are typically temporary and will subside once the exposure to the chemical stops. For instance, dermatitis caused by mild irritants is an example of a reversible effect. On the other hand, irreversible effects are permanent changes to health that cannot be undone. Some examples of irreversible health conditions caused by chemicals are asbestosis, silicosis, and cancer [5, 10, 21, 22].

6. Mechanisms of toxic effects

Chemicals can induce harmful effects or leading to diseases in humans through a variety of mechanisms.

1. Irritants such as acetone and isopropyl alcohol can cause reversible inflammatory changes in the eyes, skin, or mucous membranes of the respiratory tract. If the damage becomes irreversible, the substance is considered corrosive [7, 23].

2. Sensitizers are chemicals that can trigger an allergic response. Initially, the body may not produce any immune response upon first exposure. However, with repeated exposure, the immune system can become sensitized and then react to the allergen by causing an allergic response. For example, respiratory tract sensitizers like natural rubber latex proteins, ethylene diamine, or isocyanates can lead to asthma. On the other hand, skin sensitizers such as fragrances, formaldehyde, nickel, chromates in cement, and glutaraldehyde can cause allergic contact dermatitis [15, 21].

3. Reproductive toxins are chemicals that can hinder the reproductive capacity of both men and women. These toxins can result in various negative effects such as reduced fertility, sterility, and even spontaneous abortion [24].

4. Mutagens are chemicals that can induce mutations in the DNA of cells, potentially leading to diseases or abnormalities in future generations. For instance, mutagens like ethylene oxide and chloroform can affect cells of the reproductive system, specifically ova and sperm cells. On the other hand, mutagens such as vinyl chloride, benzene, and lead can affect cells that are not directly involved in reproductive function, such as kidney, liver, or blood cells [25].

5. Carcinogens are chemicals that can cause cancer in humans. The International Agency for Research on Cancer (IARC), which is part of the World Health Organization (WHO), has compiled a list of these carcinogens [26].

6. Genotoxicity refers to a particular form of toxicity. Genotoxic chemicals have the ability to harm and modify genetic materials found within cells, potentially leading to the development of cancer or birth defects [26].

7. Teratogens are chemicals that do not harm the mother but can lead to abnormalities, birth defects, fetal death, or developmental delays. Examples of chemical teratogens include Xylene, methyl mercury, and lead. The highest risk for these effects occurs during the 2- to 8-week stage of fetal development [24, 26].

7. Common occupational diseases caused by chemical agents

7.1 Occupational cancers

The International Agency for Research on Cancer (IARC) classifies agents into different groups based on their carcinogenicity to humans. There are five groups in total: Group 1, which includes 109 agents that are classified as carcinogenic to humans; Group 2A, which includes 65 agents that are probably carcinogenic to humans; Group 2B, which includes 275 agents that are possibly carcinogenic to humans; Group 3, which includes 503 agents that are not classifiable in terms of their carcinogenicity to humans; and Group 4, which includes agents that are probably not carcinogenic to humans [26]. **Table 2** provides a list of some proven occupational carcinogens and their associated target organs.

Many agents encountered in the workplace are considered occupational carcinogens, which can cause death and disability. Research shows that exposure to these carcinogens leads to approximately 152,000 deaths each year worldwide. Thankfully, occupational cancers can largely be prevented by improving working conditions, thus reducing the burden caused by these carcinogens [27].

Occupational cancers typically have a long latency period, meaning that there is a significant amount of time between initial exposure to the carcinogen and the development of cancer. In most cases, this period is more than 10–15 years. However, in the case of mesothelioma caused by asbestos exposure, it can take as long as 40–50 years for cancer to develop. The risk of developing cancer from occupational carcinogens is higher when exposure occurs at a younger age or when there are multiple exposures, such as smoking and asbestos exposure [26].

7.2 Occupational skin diseases

Occupational skin diseases can arise from various sources such as mechanical trauma, chemical agents, biological agents, and physical agents. Among these,

Agent	Target organ(s)
Polycyclic aromatic hydrocarbons and aromatic amines	Skin, lung, bladder
Formaldehyde	Nasal, paranasal sinuses
Ethylene oxide	Skin, lung, bladder
Benzene	Hemopoietic (blood-forming organ)
Aromatic amine carcinogens: • 4-aminibiphenyl and its nitro derivatives • B-Naphthylamine	Bladder
Metalliferous carcinogens: • Beryllium • Cadmium • Chromium • Arsenic	Lung, nasal sinuses, skin
Asbestos	Lung, larynx, ovary

Table 2.
Occupational carcinogens.

chemical agents are the primary contributors to occupational skin disease, capable of functioning as either sensitizers or irritants. Contact dermatitis is the most prevalent form of occupational skin disease, characterized by inflammation of the skin resulting from exposure to hazardous agents. This condition is classified into two primary subtypes: irritant contact dermatitis (ICD) and allergic contact dermatitis (ACD) [7, 15].

ICD is a non-immunologic inflammatory reaction of the skin, triggered by direct damage from exposure to irritants. This reaction typically occurs at the site of contact. ICD can result from acute exposure to highly irritating substances, such as acids, bases, and oxidizing or reducing agents, or from chronic, cumulative exposure to milder irritants like water, detergents, and gentle cleaning products. It is significantly more prevalent than ACD.

ACD is a delayed hypersensitivity reaction caused by dermal exposure to a skin sensitizer (allergen). Sensitization to the allergen must occur first. Upon subsequent exposure, the allergen triggers an immune response, leading to skin inflammation. Unlike ICD, the reaction is not limited to the contact site and can cause systemic effects, including rashes on other parts of the body. Workplace allergens commonly associated with ACD include industrial substances such as metals, epoxy, and acrylic resins; agrochemicals like pesticides and fertilizers; and latex.

Contact urticaria is a less common type of occupational skin disease characterized by an immediate wheal-and-flare reaction upon exposure to a contact urticant. Symptoms typically appear within 30 minutes of contact. Common triggers include latex proteins found in rubber gloves and proteinaceous raw food materials frequently handled by food preparation workers.

7.3 Occupational respiratory diseases

According to the global burden of occupational diseases study, it is estimated that there are 38,000 deaths from asthma, 30,000 deaths from pneumoconiosis, and 318,000 deaths annually from chronic obstructive pulmonary diseases [28]. **Table 3** displays a list of respiratory diseases caused by exposure to toxic chemical agents, including both acute common diseases and chronic occupational diseases [29].

Occupational asthma is a condition where the airways become narrowed and sensitive due to specific substances that are inhaled at work. A significant number of adults develop asthma as a result of exposure to these substances. There are two types

Acute occupational respiratory diseases	Chronic occupational respiratory diseases
Hypersensitivity pneumonitis	Coal workers' pneumoconiosis
Occupational asthma	Silicosis
Acute respiratory reactions to irritant gases	Asbestosis and other asbestos-related diseases (including cancers)
Acute systemic reactions to metal fumes, polymer fumes, and organic dusts	Hard metal lung disease
	Beryllium disease
	Chronic obstructive lung disease

Table 3.
Common acute and chronic occupational respiratory diseases.

of occupational asthma: immune- and non-immune-mediated. Immune-mediated asthma occurs after a period of time when a person is exposed to substances that cause an allergic reaction. Common substances that can lead to immune-mediated occupational asthma include wood dust, isocyanates, soldering, and welding fumes. Non-immune-mediated asthma, also known as reactive airway disease, can develop quickly without any delay. It is typically caused by exposure to high concentrations of chemical irritants. Accidental inhalation of irritant gases, fumes, and vapors such as chlorine can lead to reactive airway disease. The symptoms of airway irritation usually go away on their own but can sometimes persist indefinitely [23, 28].

Pneumoconiosis is a condition characterized by the fibrotic reaction of lung tissues. It is typically caused by prolonged inhalation of mineral dust. Silicosis is the most common type of pneumoconiosis worldwide, and it is caused by inhaling dust that contains crystalline silicon dioxide. Occupations with a high risk of developing this condition include polishing, quarrying, mining, stone cutting, and sandblasting [30].

8. Principles of prevention of occupational diseases due to chemical agents

Many ODs caused by specific chemical agents can be prevented by implementing three levels of prevention (**Table 4** and **Figure 1**).

Primary prevention is focused on preventing the occurrence of a disease by eliminating or preventing the causal agent from causing harm to the body. On the other hand, secondary prevention aims to detect disease in its early stages and stop its progression before it leads to clinical symptoms and signs. Tertiary prevention is meant for individuals who already have a confirmed disease and need treatment and rehabilitation to minimize complications and disabilities or to enhance their quality of life in cases where the disease is incurable. Once a case of OD resulting from chemical exposure is diagnosed, the management of the condition should extend beyond simply prescribing medication for a cure. The following steps should be taken into consideration: immediate suspension of the affected worker from any further exposure, thorough investigation and implementation of control measures to address the source of exposure, reporting the incident to relevant authorities, educating both

Primary prevention	Secondary prevention	Tertiary prevention
1. Hierarchy of controls: • Elimination • Substitution • Engineering controls to minimize exposure • Administrative controls • Personal protective equipment 2. Environmental and biological monitoring 3. Pre-placement medical examinations to identify vulnerable workers	1. Periodic medical examinations 2. Screening: early detection of exposures and effects	1. Medical treatment 2. Compensation 3. Rehabilitation

Table 4.
Prevention of occupational diseases due to chemical agents.

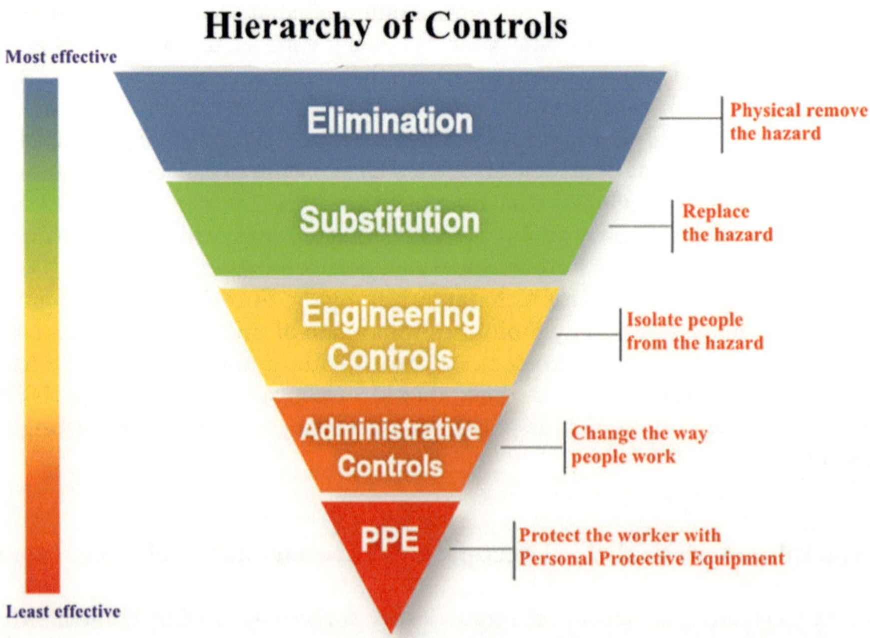

Figure 1.
The hierarchy of controls.

the patient and employer on preventive measures, identifying other workers at risk of exposure, facilitating rehabilitation efforts, conducting assessments to determine the extent of permanent disability, and providing appropriate compensation to affected workers [31, 32].

9. Risk assessment and management

Risk assessment is a critical component of occupational safety, particularly when dealing with chemical agents that pose health hazards to workers. The process of risk assessment involves the systematic identification of potential hazards, the evaluation of exposure levels, and the estimation of the likelihood and severity of adverse health effects. The primary goal of risk assessment is to provide a scientific basis for decision-making in order to reduce or eliminate risks associated with chemical exposures in the workplace.

Risk assessment is typically divided into four key steps: hazard identification, dose-response assessment, exposure assessment, and risk characterization. Each step plays a vital role in understanding the potential impact of chemical agents and in guiding the development of effective risk management strategies [33–36].

9.1 Hazard identification

Hazard identification is the first step in the risk assessment process, focusing on determining which chemicals in the workplace are capable of causing harm. This involves reviewing toxicological data, the scientific literature, and regulatory classifications to identify substances that may be hazardous. For instance, chemicals such as lead, asbestos, and benzene are well-known for their toxic effects and are classified as hazardous substances by various regulatory agencies. In addition to identifying known hazardous chemicals, this step also involves considering factors such as the chemical's physical and chemical properties, potential routes of exposure, and the presence of any vulnerable populations within the workforce. This comprehensive approach ensures that all potential risks are accounted for and that no significant hazards are overlooked [34, 35].

9.2 Dose-response assessment

The next step in the risk assessment process is dose-response assessment, which involves evaluating the relationship between the level of exposure to a chemical and the severity of the health effect it produces. This relationship is typically represented by a dose-response curve, which illustrates how increasing levels of exposure correspond to increased risks of adverse health effects.

Dose-response assessments often rely on data from animal studies, human epidemiological studies, and *in vitro* testing. These data sources provide insights into the threshold levels at which chemicals begin to cause harm, as well as the potential for severe effects at higher exposure levels. For example, the dose-response relationship for a carcinogenic substance like benzene would help determine the exposure levels that significantly increase the risk of developing cancer [12, 33].

9.3 Exposure assessment

Exposure assessment is a critical step in risk assessment that involves quantifying the levels of chemical agents to which workers are exposed. This process includes evaluating the frequency, duration, and intensity of exposure through various routes, such as inhalation, dermal contact, or ingestion.

Exposure assessment methods may include environmental monitoring, biological monitoring, and modeling techniques. Environmental monitoring involves measuring the concentration of chemicals in workplace air, while biological monitoring assesses the levels of chemicals or their metabolites in biological samples (e.g., blood, urine) from exposed workers. Modeling techniques can predict exposure levels based on factors such as the chemical's volatility, workspace ventilation, and exposure duration.

A comprehensive exposure assessment considers both average and peak exposures, as well as the potential for cumulative effects from multiple chemicals. This information is crucial for determining whether workers are at risk and for developing strategies to mitigate these exposures [22, 37].

9.4 Risk characterization

Risk characterization represents the final phase of the risk assessment process, during which data from hazard identification, dose-response analysis, and exposure evaluation are synthesized to determine the overall risk posed to workers. This step involves quantifying the likelihood of adverse health effects occurring under specific exposure conditions and determining the level of concern.

Risk characterization often involves calculating risk metrics, such as the margin of exposure (MOE) or the hazard quotient (HQ), which compare the estimated exposure levels to established safety thresholds. If the risk is deemed unacceptable, risk management actions must be implemented to reduce exposure to acceptable levels [36, 38].

9.5 Risk management strategies

Once the risk has been characterized, the next step is to implement risk management strategies aimed at controlling or eliminating chemical hazards in the workplace. The hierarchy of controls is a widely recognized framework for managing occupational risks, prioritizing measures in the following order: elimination, substitution, engineering controls, administrative controls, and personal protective equipment (PPE) [35, 39].

1. Elimination and substitution: The most effective risk management strategies involve eliminating hazardous chemicals from the workplace or substituting them with less harmful alternatives. For example, replacing a toxic solvent with a safer, water-based alternative can significantly reduce health risks.

2. Engineering controls: When elimination or substitution is not feasible, engineering controls should be implemented to reduce exposure. These controls may include ventilation systems to remove airborne contaminants, enclosures to contain hazardous processes, or automation to minimize human interaction with dangerous chemicals.

3. Administrative controls: Administrative controls focus on changing work practices and procedures to reduce the risk of exposure. Examples include rotating workers to limit the duration of exposure, implementing safe handling procedures, and providing training on the proper use of chemicals and PPE.

4. Personal protective equipment (PPE): PPE is the last line of defense and should be used when other control measures cannot fully eliminate the risk. PPE may include respirators, gloves, goggles, and protective clothing designed to shield workers from chemical exposures. However, reliance on PPE alone is not sufficient and should be complemented by other control measures.

9.6 Monitoring and evaluation

Effective risk management also requires ongoing monitoring and evaluation to ensure that control measures are working as intended. Regular environmental and biological monitoring, along with health surveillance of workers, can help identify emerging risks and guide adjustments to control strategies. Additionally, worker feedback and incident reports should be used to continually improve safety practices and reduce the potential for chemical-related occupational diseases [34].

10. Conclusion

Chemicals can exert either beneficial or harmful effects based on their application. Similar to other occupational diseases, illnesses arising from exposure to chemical hazards are largely preventable. To safeguard workers' health and safety and mitigate the adverse effects of chemical exposure, it is essential to implement control measures, with a particular emphasis on primary preventive strategies. Risk assessment and management are essential processes in occupational safety, particularly when dealing with chemical agents that pose significant health risks. By systematically identifying hazards, assessing exposures, and implementing appropriate controls, organizations can safeguard workers from the harmful effects of chemical exposure and create safer work environments. Continuous evaluation and improvement of risk management strategies are vital for adapting to new challenges and ensuring long-term occupational health and safety.

Acknowledgements

I extend my gratitude to the Publishing Process Manager, Kristina Kardum Cvitan, at IntechOpen for her invaluable guidance throughout the editorial process. While AI-powered language tools were utilized for grammar and style refinement, all content was exclusively authored by the contributors.

Conflict of interest

The authors declare no conflict of interest.

Author details

Reza Pourbabaki[1], Mohammad Amin Rajizadeh[2], Ali Faghihi Zarandi[3], Mohsen Sadeghi-Yarandi[4] and Zabiholah Damiri[5*]

1 Department of Occupational Health, School of Health, Shiraz University of Medical Sciences, Shiraz, Iran

2 Physiology Research Center, Institute of Neuropharmacology, Kerman University of Medical Sciences, Kerman, Iran

3 Department of Occupational Health Engineering, School of Public Health, Kerman University of Medical Sciences, Kerman, Iran

4 Department of Occupational Health, School of Health, Tehran University of Medical Sciences, Tehran, Iran

5 Department of Occupational Health, Faculty of Health, Ahvaz Jundishapur University of Medical Sciences, Ahvaz, Iran

*Address all correspondence to: zabiolah.damiri@gmail.com

References

[1] Pourbabaki R, Samiei S, Khadem M, kalantari S, Beigzadeh Z, Shahtaheri SJ. Antioxidant-rich products as protective agents and therapeutic factors against Chlorpyrifos hepatotoxicity – A review. Iran Occupational Health Journal. 2021;**18**(1):9

[2] Kim S et al. Investigation on combined inhalation exposure scenarios to biocidal mixtures: Biocidal and household chemical products in South Korea. Toxics. 2021;**9**(2):32

[3] Turunen E, Hiilamo H. Health effects of indebtedness: A systematic review. BMC Public Health. 2014;**14**:1-8

[4] Rantanen J, Lehtinen S, Valenti A, Iavicoli S. A global survey on occupational health services in selected international commission on occupational health (ICOH) member countries. BMC Public Health. Dec 2017;**17**:1-5

[5] Pourbabaki R et al. Role of rosemary officinalis in hepatotoxicity induced by Chlorpyrifos sub-chronic exposure in rats. Iran Occupational Health Journal. 2021;**18**(1):75-88

[6] Naafs M. Occupational diseases in the petrochemical sector and offshore upstream petroleum industry. Progress in Petrochemical Science. 2018;**2**(2):1-12

[7] Diepgen TL. Occupational skin diseases. JDDG: Journal der Deutschen Dermatologischen Gesellschaft. 2012;**10**(5):297-315

[8] Damiri Z et al. Adsorption efficacy of acetone with zeolitic imidazolate frameworks–8: A mechanistic and kinetic insight. International Journal of Environmental Analytical Chemistry. 2024;**104**(27):1-15

[9] Langman LJ, Kapur BM. Toxicology: Then and now. Clinical Biochemistry. 2006;**39**(5):498-510

[10] Borgert CJ, Fuentes C, Burgoon LD. Principles of dose-setting in toxicology studies: The importance of kinetics for ensuring human safety. Archives of Toxicology. 2021;**95**(12):3651-3664

[11] Yokoyama K. Individual susceptibility to occupational hazard. Industrial Health. 2009;**47**(5):455-458

[12] Rozman KK, Doull J, Hayes WJ Jr. Dose and time determining, and other factors influencing, toxicity. In: Hayes' Handbook of Pesticide Toxicology. 3nd ed. California: Elsevier; 2010. pp. 3-101. DOI: 10.1016/B978-0-12-374367-1.00001-X

[13] Yazid MFH, Ta GC, Mokhtar M. Classified chemicals in accordance with the globally harmonized system of classification and labeling of chemicals: Comparison of lists of the European Union, Japan, Malaysia and New Zealand. Safety and Health at Work. 2020;**11**(2):152-158

[14] Damiri Z, Jafari S, Yousefinejad S, Kazemian H. Enhanced adsorption of toluene on thermally activated ZIF-67: Characterization, performance, and modeling insights. Heliyon. 2024;**10**(9):e30745. DOI: 10.1016/j.heliyon.2024.e30745

[15] Semple S. Dermal exposure to chemicals in the workplace: Just how important is skin absorption? Occupational and Environmental Medicine. 2004;**61**(4):376-382

[16] Verma RK et al. The study of assessing the impact on environment by the noxious airborne chemicals: A review. Biointerface Research in Applied Chemistry. 2021;**11**:10844-10863

[17] Zeliger H. Human Toxicology of Chemical Mixtures. 2nd ed. Amsterdam: Elsevier; 2011

[18] Pourhossein M et al. Development of a green single drop microextraction based on deep eutectic solvent and HPLC-UV for trace residue analysis of three frequent-used pesticides. Iranian Journal of Public Health. 2023;**52**(11):2440

[19] Beigzadeh Z et al. Evaluation of pulmonary function of construction workers in Tehran city in 2017. Journal of Health and Safety at Work. 2018;**8**(4):323-332

[20] Cherrie JW et al. How important is inadvertent ingestion of hazardous substances at work? The Annals of Occupational Hygiene. 2006;**50**(7):693-704

[21] Dao A, Bernstein DI. Occupational exposure and asthma. Annals of Allergy, Asthma & Immunology. 2018;**120**(5):468-475

[22] Paustenbach DJ, Madl AK, Massarsky A. Exposure assessment. Human and Ecological Risk Assessment: Theory and Practice. 2024;**1**:157-261

[23] Patocka J, Kuca K. Irritant compounds: Respiratory irritant gases. Military Medical Science Letters. 2014;**83**(2):73-82

[24] Park C. Reproductive toxic agents in work environments and related cases in Korea. Yeungnam University Journal of Medicine. 2020;**37**(1):22-31

[25] Fishbein L. Potential carcinogenic and mutagenic industrial chemicals. I. Alkylating agents. Journal of Toxicology and Environmental Health. 1980;**6**(5-6):1133-1177

[26] International Agency for Research on Cancer. IARC monographs on the evaluation of carcinogenic risks to humans. IARC Scientific Publications. 2012;**100**:385

[27] Driscoll T et al. The global burden of disease due to occupational carcinogens. American Journal of Industrial Medicine. 2005;**48**(6):419-431

[28] Driscoll T et al. The global burden of non-malignant respiratory disease due to occupational airborne exposures. American Journal of Industrial Medicine. 2005;**48**(6):432-445

[29] Takahashi K, Koh DSQ. Textbook Of Occupational Medicine Practice. Singapore: World Scientific Publishing Company; 2011

[30] Barnes H, Glaspole I. Occupational interstitial lung diseases. Immunology and Allergy Clinics. 2023;**43**(2):323-339

[31] Lee K, Kwon HM, Cho S, Kim J, Moon I. Improvements of safety management system in Korean chemical industry after a large chemical accident. Journal of Loss Prevention in the Process Industries. 2016;**42**:6-13

[32] Piechowski LD. Evaluation of Workplace Disability. USA: Oxford University Press; 2011

[33] Cox LA Jr, Ketelslegers HB, Lewis RJ. The shape of low-concentration dose–response functions for benzene: Implications for human health risk assessment. Critical Reviews in Toxicology. 2021;**51**(2):95-116

[34] Iso I. Risk Management–Principles and Guidelines. Geneva, Switzerland: International Organization for Standardization; 2009

[35] Lyon BK, Popov G. Risk treatment strategies: Harmonizing the hierarchy of controls and inherently safer design concepts. Professional Safety. 2019;**64**(05):34-43

[36] Williams PR, Paustenbach DJ. Risk characterization. Human and Ecological Risk Assessment: Theory and Practice. 2024;**1**:263-331

[37] Samiei S et al. Protective effect of salvia officinalis extract on deltamethrin-induced hepatotoxicity in rats. Journal of Mazandaran University of Medical Sciences. 2019;**29**(178):134-140

[38] Aylward LL et al. Assessment of margin of exposure based on biomarkers in blood: An exploratory analysis. Regulatory Toxicology and Pharmacology. 2011;**61**(1):44-52

[39] Freund A. General information for controlling exposures. New Solutions: A Journal of Environmental and Occupational Health Policy. 2013;**23**:9

Chapter 2

Disaster Risk Management in Private Institutions

Bekele Getenet Tiruneh, Mengistu Abebe Messelu, Amsalu Taye and Temesgen Ayenew

Abstract

A disaster is an acute decline in society's functions, leading to extensive harm to people, property, or the environment. Based on the causes, disasters are divided into natural and man-made hazards. Significant long-term worldwide social, economic, and developmental problems may result from these circumstances, particularly if disaster risk management receives less than ideal attention. Both the public and private sectors must devote enough attention to disaster response. A continuum of prevention, readiness, response, and recovery is required for disaster risk management. Although disaster has had a significant impact in all parts of the community, engagement of the private institutions is low. Most countries were focused on the governmental institutions to prevent and provide responses to disasters. As private sectors increase in the world, the number of private employees will increase, and it needs protection and prevention of occupational safety and occupational disease.

Keywords: disaster, risk, management, private, institutions

1. Introduction

A disaster is an acute destruction of the existing environment, people, and property which is beyond the available resource. Based on the causes, it can be natural and man-made disasters. It can cause marked long-term widespread social, economic, and developmental problems which may result from these circumstances, particularly if disaster risk management is given inadequate attention [1, 2].

Despite the magnitude of disaster impact in different global regions being variable, it has an inevitable effect on societies (see **Figure 1**) [3].

A global dataset of geocoded disaster locations (GDIS) reported that 39,953 global locations were affected by 9924 disasters worldwide from 1960 to 2018 [4].

Disaster risk management is a guiding tool on which inter-sectorial contributions are made to reduce risks of disaster, severity of the loss, and duration of suffering [5].

Although disaster has had a significant impact in all parts of the community, engagement of the private institutions was low. Despite the importance of private

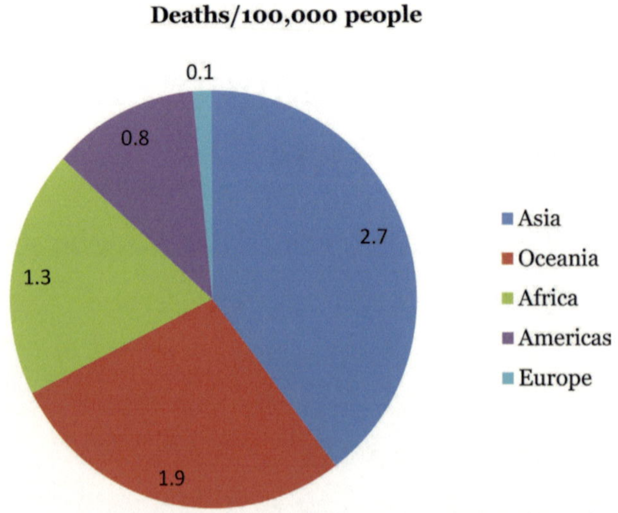

Figure 1.
Yearly average number of deaths and missing individuals per 100,000 people in different regions, 2005–2017.

sector involvement in disaster risk reduction has been recognized for decades at the international level, most countries were focused on the governmental institutions to prevent and provide a response to disaster [6].

Since 70–85% of global investment is generated by private sectors and the private capacity is expected to have strong infrastructure, institutions, human knowledge and skills, and collective attributes such as social relationships, leadership, and management, private institutions should be the major player of disaster risk management [6, 7].

Most of the buildings and infrastructures with their risks are owned by the private sector in many countries. However, the private industry had a lower contribution to disaster risk management. This indicates that private sectors missed their opportunity to provide direct benefits and co-benefits to the affected society. Mexico Case Study found that the private sector benefit-cost ratio was 4:1 regarding disaster risk management [8].

The global annual report showed that 160 million people are victims of work accidents and work-related diseases, of which 2.78 million people die of this reason. Due to direct and indirect effects, work accidents and work-related diseases resulted in a loss of 4% global domestic product (about $2.8 trillion) [9].

Natural disasters destroy $520 billion in cost of human well-being per year beyond annual asset losses [10].

Around 6.6–13% of global business risks are attributed to manmade environmental changes, loss of biodiversity, and ecosystem failure [11].

Global reports revealed that total economic losses are marked (see **Figure 2**) [12].

Private sectors are incentivized by exploring business opportunities and developing their business core model when they are active participants in disaster risk management [6, 13].

Many publications showed that disaster risk management does not have valuable concerns as a business continuity plan in private sectors [6, 14–17].

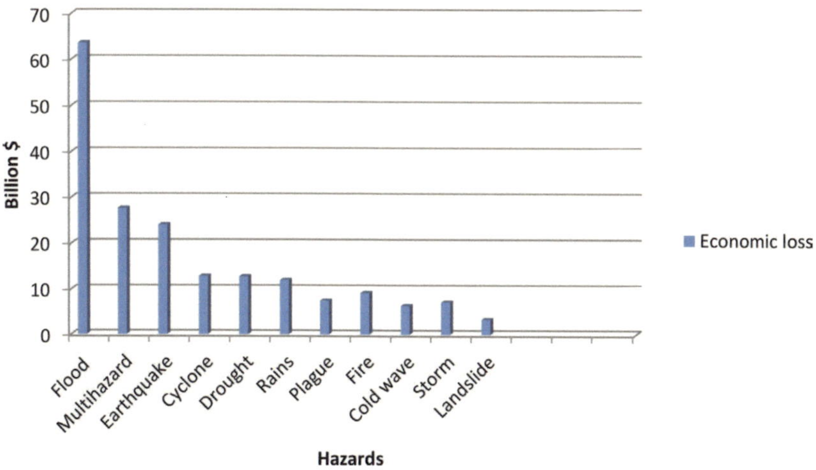

Figure 2.
Distribution of total economic loss (constant 2010 $) in 83 countries by hazard, 2005–2015.

Both the public and private sectors must devote enough attention to disaster risk management [2, 18].

Sendai Framework for Action is aimed at disaster risk management with a continuum of prevention, preparedness, response, and recovery and focused on the resilience of communities, and health and social systems. This framework also suggests the integration of public and private sectors with affected communities [19].

The private sector is also encouraged to integrate disaster risk management into its business models [20].

Through responsible actions and partnerships that have the potential to capitalize on both organizations' core competencies, improve disaster prevention, raise awareness of the corporate brand, and contribute to disaster risk management and mitigation, the private sector can assist the public sector by providing resources and expertise in disaster risk management [21].

There are two sides to the relationship between disaster and private investment: (1) Disaster can affect private investment. (2) Private investment can increase the risk of disaster [14].

Protection of employees and occupational activity in risky zones are included in corporate social responsibility (CSR) related to disaster risk management [14].

Besides governments and international organizations, private sector engagement in disaster risk management is encouraged by international business institutions and economic forums. Economic globalization has increased business productivity and reduced poverty with an associated risk of natural disasters [22].

Most private institutions did not understand their possibilities and advantages during disaster risk management participation. Companies have to build corporate culture and disaster response codes and policies for their survival, assets, employees, and overall community resilience [11, 23].

Workplace safety is the common responsibility that binds business sectors and countries regarding disaster risk management [24].

This chapter summarized different international, national, and regional level literature about the engagement of private institutions in disaster risk management.

2. Literatures review

As the modern global economy is mainly dependent on private businesses, we tried to organize the different levels of published literature focused on private sector involvement in disaster risk management.

A disaster is a severe, acute decline in societal functioning that overwhelms the affected areas to handle their resources and needs external assistance [25].

"Since 1990, disasters resulted in the loss of about 1.6 million lives worldwide or about 65,000 people every year and caused trillions of dollars' worth of losses in associated damages." A developing country's achievement can be drastically altered by disasters, which can also undermine years of progress [2].

This significant destruction is also reported by other global studies (see **Figure 3**) [3].

Around 6.6–13% of global business risks are attributed to manmade environmental changes, loss of biodiversity, and ecosystem failure [11].

Natural disasters destroy $520 billion in cost of human well-being per year beyond annual asset losses [10].

According to global estimates, 18% of the deaths attributable to occupational risks are caused by workplace injuries [26].

In recent years, natural disasters have occurred frequently, and human and economic problems have worsened. Households, communities, and low-level businesses are significantly affected by such disasters [10]. These disasters affected all parts of the world (**see Table 1**) [12].

The subject of emergency and disaster management still lacks modern management ideas and understanding. A modern perspective on disaster management emphasizes the creative and modern aspects of the process while encouraging broader participation from individuals and the public. Even if the recent COVID-19 pandemic has had a lot of negative effects, it has positively impacted how the conventional

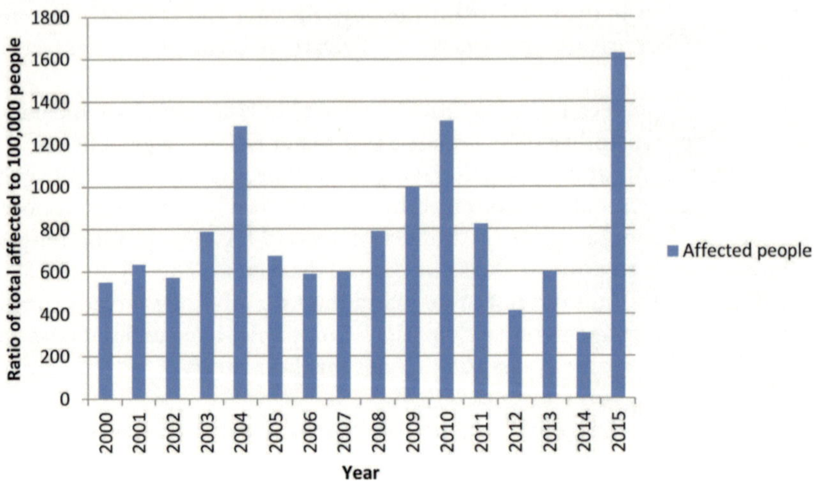

Figure 3.
Number of people affected in Sendai framework monitor system 83 countries with 2000–2015 data.

Regions	Occurrence (%)	Deaths (%)	Affected (%)	Economic loss (%)
Africa	21.6	17.1	13.7	10.8
Europe	6.0	0.8	1.2	7.0
Americas	46.4	11.9	32.8	39.1
Asia	22.9	69.7	52.2	42.0
Oceania	3.0	0.5	0.2	1.0

Table 1.
Percentage of disaster occurrences and impacts in different regions, 2005–2015.

disaster management cycle is used all over the world. Because the conventional cycle of disaster management is procedural, it needs to incorporate more value-based techniques and modern management theory [27].

The application of Artificial intelligence should be practiced in four phases of disaster management (preparedness, mitigation, response, and recovery) rather than the response phase only. It is also suggested that future research have to address the challenges of AI techniques to inspire professional communities [28].

Aside from the COVID-19 pandemic, recent years have been characterized primarily by climate-related disasters, according to data gathered by the Emergency Events Database (EM-DAT). One such year was the warmest on record. Disasters have major and frequently disastrous societal effects in addition to human casualties, such as economic losses. The severe and frequently catastrophic effects of disasters have been better handled because of recent advancements in artificial intelligence (AI), particularly in machine learning and deep learning [29].

To combat natural catastrophes, manage associated risks, and organize emergency responses, data from social media, drones, multimedia, and search engines can be utilized [30].

A study conducted in eight European countries (Belgium, Estonia, Finland, Germany, Hungary, Italy, Norway, and Sweden) revealed that there was a significant difference between these countries in terms of reduction strategies, an ontology of vulnerability, and its sources and resource allocation activities. A heuristic model can clarify the conceptual difference and variable understanding of vulnerability along with human agency's strong public-private relation. This enables to guide risk analysis and future planning for early adaptation of different disasters [31].

Maintaining public health and the economic advancement of any country in the linked world depends on ensuring global health security. At the national and international levels, emergency preparedness is seen as the key to managing the growing public health concerns. Predictive information systems, which rely on regular surveillance, disease modeling, and forecasting, are also essential for developing policies and involving the community in the identification, mitigation, and response to possible health risks. Thus, accurate and early predictions of these unfortunate occurrences could facilitate quick and efficient public health reactions and mitigation initiatives. This analysis centers on public health surveillance, epidemiological modeling, and capacity-building strategies as key components of emergency preparedness. Under the One Health paradigm, global coordination and capacity building, finance, and commitment at the national and international levels are essential to effectively addressing challenges to global public health [32].

Scholars showed the importance of a strong linkage between global risk management and the influential international organization (World Economic Forum) for sustainable, safe, inclusive, and resilient development [33].

In addition to highlighting the importance of cooperation and coordination in readiness and response, the reports from 11 Sub-Saharan African and South Asian nations also identified four critical components that define and facilitate efficient coordination. Initially, there must be fair gender representation in the coordination process, bringing together various government sectors and levels as well as stakeholders from the business, public, and development sectors, as well as local leaders. The availability of coordination structures and regular meeting venues; the importance of enhancing already-existing coordination mechanisms; the continued operation of coordination bodies both before and after crises; and the clear roles, mandates, and sufficient authority are among the second-tier structural aspects of coordination bodies that must be considered. Third, organizations responsible for coordination require sufficient capacity, including staff, funding, communication infrastructure, and other resources, and learning from previous emergencies. Fourth, effective coordination is supported by high-level political leadership and incentives for collaboration. Country experience also highlighted interactions between these components, and with the wider health system and governance architecture, pointing to the need to consider coordination as part of a complex adaptive system [34].

One study examined a channel through which corporate social responsibility affects firm performance. More specifically, it modeled the mediating role of enterprise risk management between corporate social responsibility and firm performance. Drawing on the stakeholder theory and using a large sample of 1021 Asia Pacific firms throughout 2006–2016, it showed that corporate social responsibility is positively associated with firm performance. The result suggested that corporate social responsibility is linked to enterprise risk management [35].

Disasters are not external events to development rather they are the result of development activity. So the Global Assessment Report (GAR) recommends integration has to be applied to all sectorial development plans [36].

Disaster risk management is a guiding tool on which inter-sectorial contributions are made to reduce risks of disaster, severity of the loss, and duration of suffering [5].

As part of shaping future production initiatives, leaders of business sectors and industries must ensure their inclusive and continued economic growth. Technology innovation and distribution, concerned common assets, and responsible workforce strategies enable economic growth more advanced.

If the production sector provides demand-oriented products and services that improve quality of life while reducing consumption of natural resources as well as minimizing the risk of toxic materials, pollutants, and wastes, the sector is called a "sustainable production sector." Government, business sectors and civil society need to have clear conversations to strengthen collaboration between industrialization and attainment of sustainable development goals and, ultimately to create action-oriented projects to solve problems and seek optimal benefits [11].

If corporate social responsibility in disaster risk management is realized as sectorial risk management, proactive measures must be taken for natural disasters. This is a collaborative effort with other stakeholders to minimize the impact of natural disasters [37].

In recent years, the private sector has been engaged in humanitarian activity by collaborating with the humanitarian community and innovative sectors. Private enterprises are progressively being viewed as a substitute for foreign aid organizations, especially in middle-income, "emerging," and state-capitalist economies, as well as in nations that are cautious about their internal affairs. As companies have been more involved in humanitarian activity, entire aspects of it, like cash transfers, telecommunications, and logistics, have changed [38].

There will be a growing number of emergencies in middle-income countries that have strong local business sectors and are resistant to wider international aid efforts. Businesses, which are often concentrated in cities, now have more chances due to the quickening pace of urbanization and the more urban nature of humanitarian crises. Future crises will frequently call for solutions that go beyond traditional assistance agency strategies and the need for an increasing degree of technical proficiency. When humanitarian organizations work to adapt to new kinds of crises, the private sector is thought to offer the best potential solution to the problem of humanitarian capacity [38].

The main motivation behind the private sector's involvement in emergency response has been to employ resources to help lessen suffering and to prioritize the well-being of those affected. This is especially true for local and national businesses, where doing good deeds is frequently seen as a moral, religious, or national obligation. Business executives are becoming more familiar with affected individuals by global media, information and communications technology, and the globalization of commerce. These individuals include suppliers, customers, clients, and coworkers. As a result, companies are involved in disaster reduction more often than they were in earlier decades [38].

Aid organizations can assist businesses in understanding how to support humanitarian aims by creating a logical collection of professional and easily accessible information concerning humanitarian action, such as publications, training materials, podcasts, or videos. It will be crucial to work with communications, public relations, and new media firms to make sure that these illustrative materials are comprehensible and appealing to a broad audience that extends beyond corporate social responsibility departments of organizations [38].

If individuals are well-informed and motivated in disaster prevention and restoration, disasters can be significantly decreased. This necessitates gathering, compiling, and disseminating pertinent knowledge and information on hazards, vulnerabilities, and capacities [39].

Most buildings and a substantial amount of the infrastructure that is at risk are owned by the private sector in most countries. The private sector, on the other hand, lags well behind the public sector in terms of investment in disaster risk management. This means that companies miss the direct benefits of disaster risk management and co-benefits to the company and society. These co-benefits include strategies for reducing production costs, enhancing worker health, and promoting overall economic stability. The Mexico Case Study found that the private sector benefit-cost ratio was 4:1 regarding disaster risk management [8].

Most private businesses are still unaware of the benefits, opportunities, and possibilities of taking part in disaster risk reduction activities. The current studies showed that, to facilitate this process, there must be functioning public institutions with designated coordinating bodies, access to finance, appropriate and simple-to-understand rules and regulations, and information sharing [11].

The necessity of multi-stakeholder participation in disaster management was also emphasized by the Hyogo Framework for Action (HFA), which was approved by 168 nations at the UN World Conference on Disaster Reduction in 2005. The statement called "the full commitment and involvement of all actors concerned including governments, regional and international organizations, and civil society including volunteers, the private sector, and the scientific community" [40].

Sendai framework reported the magnitude of life loss due to different accidents as shown in (**Figure 4**) [3].

Significant efforts have been made since 2015 to put the Sendai Framework into practice by an increasing number of stakeholders from various sectors, scales, and geographic locations. The Sendai Framework for Disaster Risk Reduction 2015–2030 highlights that risk is everyone's concern and makes it clear that participation from institutions across the state and society as a whole is required [41].

The risk of both small- and large-scale, frequent and infrequent, rapid and slow-onset disasters caused by natural or man-made hazards, as well as associated environmental, technical, and biological hazards and risks, was covered under the Sendai Framework for Disaster Risk Reduction 2015–2030. It seeks to provide guidance for the multi-hazard management of risks in development across all sectors and at all levels [36].

By implementing integrated and inclusive economic, structural, legal, social, health, cultural, educational, environmental, technological, political, and institutional measures that prevent and reduce hazard exposure and vulnerability to disasters, increase preparedness for response and recovery, and ultimately strengthen resilience. One of the goals of the Sendai Framework is to prevent new disasters and reduce existing ones [36].

The goal of the Sendai framework 2015–2030 is to significantly lower the risk of disasters, the number of fatalities, the loss of livelihoods, health, and the economic, physical, social, cultural, and environmental assets of people, businesses, communities, and nations. Additionally, it seeks to manage disasters from a multi-risk and multi-sectorial perspective, addressing hazards of any magnitude, regularity, sudden or gradual progression, and origin. The reduction of disaster risk necessitates a shared responsibility between national and local governments as well as other interested sectors. As a result, the process calls for the cooperation and dedication of the entire society, along with a distinct division of roles between the public and private sectors [19].

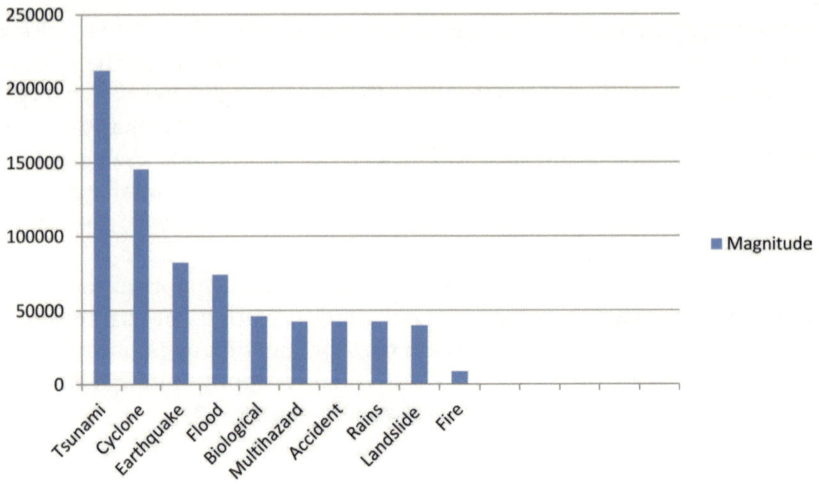

Figure 4.
Hazard distribution of mortality 1997–2017, for all countries in the Sendai framework monitoring system.

Encouraging people to invest in structural and non-structural disaster risk reduction and prevention is crucial for improving the social, cultural, health, and economic resilience of individuals, communities, nations, and their resources, as well as the environment. These have the potential to spur innovation, expansion, and job creation. These affordable actions are essential for preserving life, preventing and minimizing losses, and ensuring fast recovery and rehabilitation [36].

Business operations are disrupted by disasters that cause damage to offices, factories, and other resources and infrastructure. Physical asset destruction decreased operational performance, and disturbance to personnel and the workplace is one of these direct effects. Damage to ports, airports, transportation and energy networks, or residential areas of personnel indirectly disrupts operations and increases costs. In the current globalized pattern, even companies located in safety must deal with natural disasters that strike partners and suppliers in other parts of the world. Companies, industries, and nations experience these indirect effects because of the globalization of value chains and marketplaces. As a result, the private sector needs to plan to minimize these effects and damages. The private sector should be involved in disaster risk management for reasons other than the effects of disasters on enterprises and the world economy [42, 43].

Studies have indicated that increased regional economies do not result in decreased disaster losses or decreased human exposure to disasters [44, 45].

It's interesting to note that company investments typically increase the risk of disaster for companies, their supply chains, and the communities where they operate [22].

Due to accessible export markets and reduced labor expenses, companies frequently locate in developing countries that are more disaster-prone due to high population density and inadequate safety precautions. These places are vulnerable to disaster events that can cause enormous harm, including increased poverty, decreased productivity, and asset destruction. This eventually becomes a vicious cycle that restricts development activities and procedures. In certain instances, the private sector's choices, preparations, and actions generate and maintain these elevated risks. Consequently, the private sector bears the responsibility of mitigating disaster risks to which it may have contributed and enhancing the resilience of businesses and communities. The private sector's wealth of resources, knowledge, and technological capabilities is its greatest asset. This industry should do everything in its power to safeguard social security and private companies. It is necessary to deploy these skills and abilities for cooperative disaster risk reduction initiatives. To achieve this, businesses need to think about security "outside the fence," as well as how they might help local communities coordinate and integrate disaster risk management [46].

In addition to natural disasters and work-related disasters, conflict and violence resulted in displacement of local communities (see **Table 2**) [3].

Even while the private sector has contributed in various ways and during numerous disasters, most of these contributions are made during the reaction stage rather than over long-term contributions. Encouraging multi-stakeholder engagement and strong government leadership are essential for increasing private sector enterprises' long-term participation. In addition to governments and international organizations, business, and economic forums and institutions have also emphasized the significance of private sector participation in disaster recovery and rehabilitation. Economic globalization has decreased poverty and increased corporate productivity and efficiency, but these benefits have come at the expense of increased vulnerability to the negative effects of natural disasters [22].

Year	Disaster (Million)	Conflict (Million)
2008	36.5	4.6
2009	16.7	6.5
2010	42.4	2.9
2011	15	3.5
2012	32.4	6.6
2013	22.1	8.2
2014	19.1	11
2015	19.2	8.6
2016	24.2	6.9
2017	18.8	11.8

Table 2.
New displacement due to disasters and conflict, 2008–2017.

Innovative activities in disaster management can benefit a business in the following ways:

1. Safeguard its own operations, supply chain, clients, and employees.

2. Establish a positive reputation and act responsibly.

3. Strengthen partnership with the government.

4. Influence stakeholder perception.

5. Improve staff retention and motivation.

6. Offer fresh commercial prospects that generate mutual benefit.

In addition, the World Economic Forum (WEF) (2008) highlighted four areas of opportunity where the private sector can help create disaster resilience for communities and businesses:

1. Keeping an eye on hazards and conveying risk via forecasts and alerts.

2. Socio-physical strengthening via sea walls and dams, as well as supply chain adaptability.

3. Using disaster insurance pools to share financial risk.

4. Preparing for disasters via staff training, GIS, flood management, etc.

Four industrial communities were found to be the most active in constructing resilience to address these areas: ICT and Telecom, Engineering and Construction, Utilities and Transportation, and Insurers and Reinsurers [11].

Ensuring company continuity both during and after disasters and being ready for a wide range of disruptions in advance are the main incentives for the private sector to participate in disaster management. The private sector can also make a greater contribution by investigating business prospects and developing their fundamental business models.

There are five identified methods for engaging the private sector:

1. Direct support to communities.

2. Preparedness for own business for disasters.

3. Creation of innovative products grounded in business, technology, and knowledge.

4. Cooperative project as implementer involving NGOs, governments, and international organizations.

5. The establishment of trusts, NGOs, and private foundations.

Since the third and fourth models in particular call for close cooperation and support from stakeholders, other stakeholders must work to encourage the private sector to participate in their projects and offer advice and information when needed to increase the private sector's involvement. Collaboration between multiple stakeholders is essential to promoting private sector involvement.

The private sector plays a critical role in disaster risk management in the current global economy.

The private sector must contribute to the protection of international supply chains in addition to safeguarding its investments and companies to guarantee continuous operations and production both during and after disasters. The private sector must comprehend the potential for DRR activities to generate commercial opportunities and broaden company markets. Meanwhile, private sector companies need to be included as important players in program development and planning processes, not simply donors, according to other stakeholders like governments, non-governmental organizations, and academic institutions [6].

The Third UN World Conference for Disaster Risk Reduction in 2015 featured a gathering of the business sector community, organized by UNISDR. The 300-person business sector delegation participated on panels, acted as moderators, and presented private sector approaches to lower the risk of disaster. The realization of the private sector's crucial role in accomplishing the objectives of the Sendai Framework for Disaster Risk Reduction 2015–2030 was one of the results of the efforts made both before and during the World Conference. This is clear from the 35 times the private sector is mentioned in the Sendai Framework [19].

The private sector has begun to make further investments in initiatives to minimize the vulnerabilities of the local areas where their employee resides, in addition to striving to minimize the potential effects of catastrophes on their operations. It is also suggested for the private sector to incorporate DRM into their business plans [41].

The important concerns of engagement, motivation, and policy need to be addressed to further promote private sector involvement in disaster risk reduction. These are thought to be successful means of involving the private sector [6].

The Philippine Disaster Resilience Foundation (the world's first private sector-operated self-sufficient Emergency Operations Centre) has promoted a comprehensive approach to disaster risk management (DRM), as evidenced by its shifting priorities from a "reactive" emphasis on disaster recovery processes to "proactive" disaster preparedness and recovery [47, 48].

The establishment of the UNISDR Business Sector Alliance for Disaster Resilient Societies (ARISE) in November marked a significant milestone following the success of the business sector's input at the World Conference in March 2015 and in response to the call made in the Sendai Framework. Combining the efforts of UNISDR's business Sector Advisory Group, Private Sector Partnership, and ARISE Initiative, this signified a strengthening of UNISDR's approach to the business sector. ARISE was created as a means for the private sector to meet the goals outlined in the Sendai Framework. Additionally, ARISE assisted educational institutions, training facilities and programs, and business associations in enhancing their business risk management curricula. There is now a postgraduate diploma in urban disaster resilience offered by Florida International University. Furthermore, a one-day course for business owners or operators has been designed, and two training institutions in Chile and Colombia have been identified as prototype partners for disaster risk management training, specifically for small and medium-sized businesses [19].

To improve their disaster and climate risk management, 222 firms and organizations in seven countries were trained using the "Make Your Business Disaster and Climate Resilient" tool in 2015. Cost-sharing arrangements were used to operate the courses, with the private sector organizations offering the tools needed to conduct the training, which was conducted with assistance from regional partners in Fiji, the Republic of Korea, the Philippines, Georgia, Indonesia, Jordan, and Vietnam.

Additionally, they covered a wide range of industries, including manufacturing, public sector, tourism, water and energy, transportation and logistics, education, real estate developers, retail, and fishing/farming sectors. About 85% of the participating companies and organizations employed one hundred people or more [19].

The Hyogo Framework for Action 2015–2030 encourages gender and cultural sensitivity training as essential elements of education and training for disaster risk reduction, as well as the implementation of local risk assessment and disaster preparedness programs in schools and higher education institutions. It also encourages the private sector to cultivate a culture of disaster prevention by placing more emphasis on and funding pre-disaster activities like risk assessments and early warning systems. These partnerships with the public sector aim to better involve the private sector in disaster risk reduction activities [19, 39].

The Hyogo Action Framework, 2015–2030 encourages the integration of disaster risk reduction as a fundamental component of the United Nations Decade of Education for Sustainable Development and encourages the inclusion of disaster risk reduction knowledge in pertinent sections of school curricula at all levels and the use of other formal and informal channels to reach youth and children with information [39].

The mitigation of disaster risk should be systematically addressed at all grade levels and throughout the curriculum. Prevention, mitigation, vulnerability, and resilience building must all be taken into consideration in addition to the fundamental science of dangers and safety precautions. To equip teachers to effectively teach disaster risk reduction curricula, they must get training in both disaster and hazard-related subjects [49].

Postgraduate students at a private dental school in India participated in a study where they scored highly on attitude but poorly on knowledge and behavior related to disaster management. This study has policy implications for disaster management in India and emphasizes the need for modifications to the curriculum in dental education [50].

A study conducted in Saudi Arabian hospitals (December 2015–April 2016) revealed that most of the deficiencies, especially regarding hospital personnel education, training, and oversight regarding their readiness for disaster emergencies. Few hospitals had practiced staff and patient evacuation in the past 12 months, few had done a casualty exercise, and no hospital had done an unannounced exercise in the previous year [17].

In a study done in Ethiopian private hospitals, most of the healthcare workers had poor levels of knowledge and practice in disaster risk management [16].

According to an Iranian survey, the average level of disaster readiness across all hospitals was 59.5%; teaching hospitals scored 62.2%, while private hospitals scored 55% [15].

A study done in Japan emphasized the importance of 4P (Public-Private-People Partnership) to tackle the triple disaster (radiation disasters, Nuclear Power Plant accident, and the Great East Japan earthquake) and COVID-19 pandemic [51].

Many authors suggest that new forms of cooperation between private and public sectors can help countries finance disaster risks [6].

Disasters have pushed private enterprises to reevaluate their position and take social responsibility and strategy into account while engaging in humanitarian work. Despite the risks, these corporations think that by improving as corporate citizens, they may benefit society as well as their business. However, humanitarian organizations also acknowledge that the private sector can provide resources and expertise, as well as opportunities to enhance their impact on society through collaboration and responsible actions that further facilitate the sharing of best practices and knowledge [6].

A study conducted in Japan provided a clear explanation of the bottom-up strategy developed by certain private-sector physicians to foster citywide cooperation for disaster planning. To establish coordination mechanisms, their initial objective was to create a combined exercise that included all municipal health facilities and workers. They then planned to gradually increase the drill's degree of practice to enhance each hospital's capabilities. Since the majority of private practitioners belonged to local medical, dental, and pharmaceutical associations, the project combined these groups to engage not just hospital workers but also healthcare personnel in their private practices [52].

To empower and include all stakeholders, to lay the groundwork for gender equality, and to include individuals and groups who are more exposed to and vulnerable to the effects of disasters, frameworks like Sendai are essential [41].

Six American cities participated in a study on disaster risk reduction and the private sector. The main conclusions, derived from responses to almost 1200 surveys, were as follows:

1. 56% of respondents do not have a business continuity plan in place.

2. 36.5% of businesses stated that other priorities take precedence over a business continuity plan.

3. In addition to financial constraints, the lack of protection in the private sector is caused by issues that are still poorly understood, such as avoidance, the justification of competing priorities, limited decision-making, and concerns about accountability.

There are two sides to the interaction between disaster risks and private investments. Disasters can have an impact on private investments, and they can also create or increase the risks of disasters.

Several activities fall under the category of corporate social responsibility related to disaster risk reduction, including protection of employees and conducting business in dangerous areas [14].

Provinces with large economies or industrial areas tend to have a private sector predominance when it comes to disaster management. Relationships frequently take the form of mutual dependence. For instance, government organizations are not adequate to handle major disasters like chemical and hazardous material-related incidents. As a result, many local administrators enter into memorandums of agreement with the private sector to allow the latter to provide some technical support when needed, such as in complex situations requiring emergency professionals and professional protocol that locals might not be able to handle [53].

The adoption of practices typical of occupational risk management ought to be part of a revised model of Russia's Health, Safety, and Environment Management System. The creation and application of the new model enable the shift from the approach of responding to the reality of injuries or occupational diseases that have already occurred to the process of developing and implementing preventative measures against accidents and for preserving the health of employees [54].

3. Conclusion

Studies conducted by international, national, and regional levels and global leaders encouraged the active participation of private sectors in disaster risk management.

It is concluded that the private sector should be highly involved in all parts of disaster risk management (prevention, emergency management, restoration, recovery) as it has a significant contribution to the global economy, employee engagement, and increased risk of disaster vulnerability. Corporate social responsibility promotes participation of private investment in the community, environment, and its employees. Besides, the public sectors are encouraged to share continuous information and

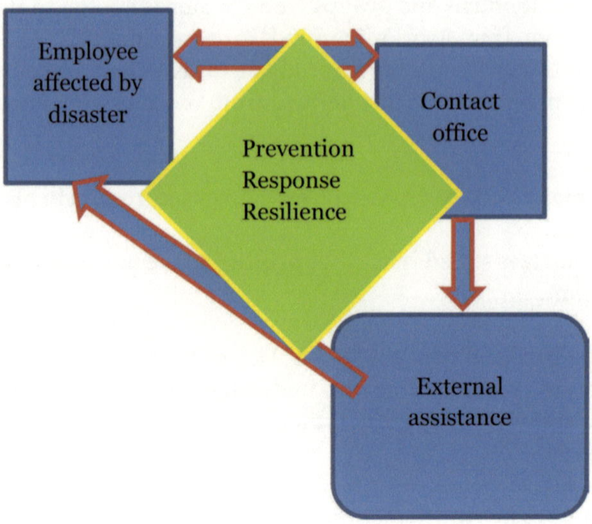

Figure 5.
Road map of employee during disaster in their workplace.

incentives. We suggested future studies focus on the contemporary view of disaster risk management to effectively utilize advanced technologies and experienced professional experts.

Every employee should get insurance, training on disaster risk management, and routine drills (every 6 months) in the workplace.

Disaster is inevitable with human development activities and once it happens, the diagram below is the guide on how employees should follow and ask the employer to be visible during the event (see **Figure 5**).

Acknowledgements

The authors acknowledge IntechOpen for giving us this chance.

Conflict of interest

The authors declare that there is no conflict of interest.

Author details

Bekele Getenet Tiruneh*, Mengistu Abebe Messelu, Amsalu Taye and Temesgen Ayenew
Debre Markos University, Debre Markos, Ethiopia

*Address all correspondence to: bekeleget12@gmail.com; bekele_getnet@dmu.edu.et

References

[1] Waganew W, Azazh A. Disaster medical assistant team establishment and the disaster response experience of Ethiopia. The Ethiopian Journal of Health Development. 2021;**35**(4):1-6

[2] Organization WH. Consultation on the Health Emergency Risk Management Framework and Improving Public Health Preparedness: Meeting Report, WHO Headquarters, Geneva, Switzerland, 21-23 November 2012. Geneva, Switzerland: World Health Organization; 2013

[3] McGlade J, Bankoff G, Abrahams J, Cooper-Knock S, Cotecchia F, Desanker P, et al. Global Assessment Report on Disaster Risk Reduction 2019. New York, USA: UN Office for Disaster Risk Reduction; 2019

[4] Rosvold EL, Buhaug H. GDIS, a global dataset of geocoded disaster locations. Scientific Data. 2021;**8**(1):61

[5] Eyerkaufer ML, Lima FS, Goncalves MB. Public and private partnership in disaster risk management. Jamba. 2016;**8**(1):277

[6] Izumi T, Shaw R. Overview and introduction of the private sector's role in disaster management. In: Disaster Management and Private Sectors: Challenges and Potentials. Japan: Springer; 2015. pp. 1-10

[7] Bopape M, Nemakonde LD, Fourie K. Private companies and community collaboration: Towards building disaster resilience in Diepsloot, Johannesburg, South Africa. Jàmbá: Journal of Disaster Risk Studies. 2021;**13**(1):1-11

[8] Rose A. Capturing the co-Benefits of Disaster Risk Management on the Private Sector Side. Vol. 7634. California, USA: World Bank Policy Research Working Paper; 2016

[9] Organization IL. The Prevention of Occupational Diseases. Geneva, Switzerland: International Labour Organization; 2013

[10] Kull D, Gitay H, Bettencourt S, Reid R, Simpson A, McCall K. Building resilience: World bank group experience in climate and disaster resilient development. In: Climate Change Adaptation Strategies–An Upstream-Downstream Perspective. Switzerland: Springer; 2016. pp. 255-270

[11] Fekete BM, Revenga C, Todd M. The Global Risks Report 2018 13th Edition. Vol. 31(1). Geneva: World Economic Forum; 2018, 2009. pp. 50-67. Agricultural Economics. Available from: http://www3.weforum.org/docs/WEF_GRR18_Report.pdf

[12] Aronsson-Storrier M. UN Office for Disaster Risk Reduction. Yearbook of International Disaster Law Online. Cambridge, UK: UN Office for Disaster Risk Reduction. 2022;**3**(1):417-423

[13] Mavrodieva AV, Shaw R. Enabling private sector engagement in disaster resilience in South and East Asia. Risk, Hazards & Crisis in Public Policy. 2019;**10**(4):466-483

[14] Sarmiento JP, Hoberman G, Ilcheva M, Asgary A, Majano AM, Poggione S, et al. Private sector and disaster risk reduction: The cases of Bogota, Miami, Kingston, San Jose, Santiago, and Vancouver. International Journal of Disaster Risk Reduction. 2015;**14**:225-237

[15] Mahdaviazad H, Abdolahifar GR. Assessing hospital disaster preparedness

in Shiraz, Iran 2011: Teaching versus private hospitals. American Journal of Disaster Medicine. 2013;**8**(1):65-73

[16] Getenet B, Waganew W, Keney D, Yesuf A. Knowledge, attitude and practices of frontline health care workers to disaster risk management in private general hospitals in Addis Ababa, Ethiopia: Multicenter cross-sectional study. Ethiopian Journal of Health Sciences. 2023;**33**(5):795-804

[17] Bin Shalhoub AA, Khan AA, Alaska YA. Evaluation of disaster preparedness for mass casualty incidents in private hospitals in Central Saudi Arabia. Saudi Medical Journal. 2017;**38**(3):302-306

[18] Djalante R, Thomalla F, Sinapoy MS, Carnegie M. Building resilience to natural hazards in Indonesia: Progress and challenges in implementing the Hyogo framework for action. Natural Hazards. 2012;**62**:779-803

[19] Aitsi-Selmi A, Egawa S, Sasaki H, Wannous C, Murray V. The Sendai framework for disaster risk reduction: Renewing the global commitment to people's resilience, health, and well-being. International Journal of Disaster Risk Science. 2015;**6**:164-176

[20] Aronsson-Storrier M, UN Office for Disaster Risk Reduction. Yearbook of International Disaster Law Online. Vol. 2(1). New York, USA: UN Office for Disaster Risk Reduction; 2021. pp. 377-382

[21] Tomasini RM, Van Wassenhove LN. From preparedness to partnerships: Case study research on humanitarian logistics. International Transactions in Operational Research. 2009;**16**(5):549-559

[22] Sharma B. Contextualising CSR in Asia: Corporate Social Responsibility in Asian Economies. Singapore: Lien Centre for Social Innovation; 2013

[23] Sierra L, Zorio A, García-Benau MA. Sustainable development and assurance of corporate social responsibility reports published by Ibex-35 companies. Corporate Social Responsibility and Environmental Management. 2013;**20**(6):359-370

[24] Soerjaman KV, Blanpain SPDR, Rombouts L. Employers' Liability for Damage Caused by his Employee. Netherlands: University of Tilburg; 2013

[25] Tintinalli JE, Stapczynski JS, Ma OJ, Cline D, Meckler GD, Yealy DM. Tintinalli's Emergency Medicine: A Comprehensive Study Guide. New York: McGraw-Hill Education; 2016

[26] Rushton L. The global burden of occupational disease. Current Environmental Health Reports. 2017;**4**:340-348

[27] Sawalha IH. A contemporary perspective on the disaster management cycle. Foresight. 2020;**22**(4):469-482

[28] Sun W, Bocchini P, Davison BD. Applications of artificial intelligence for disaster management. Natural Hazards. 2020;**103**(3):2631-2689

[29] Linardos V, Drakaki M, Tzionas P, Karnavas YL. Machine learning in disaster management: Recent developments in methods and applications. Machine Learning and Knowledge Extraction. 2022;**4**(2):446-473

[30] Munawar HS, Qayyum S, Ullah F, Sepasgozar S. Big data and its applications in smart real estate and the disaster management life cycle: A systematic analysis. Big Data and Cognitive Computing. 2020;**4**(2):4

[31] Orru K, Hansson S, Gabel F, Tammpuu P, Krüger M, Savadori L, et al. Approaches to 'vulnerability' in eight European disaster management systems. Disasters. 2022;**46**(3):742-767

[32] Bedi JS, Vijay D, Dhaka P, Gill JPS, Barbuddhe SB. Emergency preparedness for public health threats, surveillance, modelling & forecasting. Indian Journal of Medical Research. 2021;**153**(3):287-298

[33] Sharma S, Soederberg S. Redesigning the business of development: The case of the world economic forum and global risk management. Review of International Political Economy. 2020;**27**(4):828-854

[34] Gooding K, Bertone MP, Loffreda G, Witter S. How can we strengthen partnership and coordination for health system emergency preparedness and response? Findings from a synthesis of experience across countries facing shocks. BMC Health Services Research. 2022;**22**(1):1441

[35] Naseem T, Shahzad F, Asim GA, Rehman IU, Nawaz F. Corporate social responsibility engagement and firm performance in Asia Pacific: The role of enterprise risk management. Corporate Social Responsibility and Environmental Management. 2020;**27**(2):501-513

[36] Pearson L, Pelling M. The UN Sendai framework for disaster risk reduction 2015-2030: Negotiation process and prospects for science and practice. Journal of Extreme Events. 2015;**2**(01):1571001

[37] Hishan S, Ramakrishnan S, Manokaran K, Vaicondam Y. Corporate social responsibility for natural disaster: A new method for organizational risk management. Journal of Advanced Research in Dynamical and Control Systems. 2020;**12**(1):111-115

[38] Drummond J, Crawford N. HPG. 2014;**02**:1-37

[39] United Nations. A/CONF. 206/6. Strasbourg, France: Report of the World Conference on Disaster Reduction; 2005

[40] Petal M, Izadkhah YO. Concept note: Formal and informal education for disaster risk reduction. In: Proceedings of the International Conference on School Safety, Islamabad, Pakistan. Geneva, Switzerland: Citeseer; 2008

[41] Chmutina K, Von Meding J, Bosher L. Language matters: Dangers of the "natural disaster" misnomer. In: Global Assessment Report on Disaster Risk Reduction (GAR 2019). New York, USA: Global Assessment Report 2019; 2019

[42] De Bono A. Global Exposure Database for GAR 2013. Geneva, Switzerland: UNISDR; 2013. p. 39

[43] Corner EDs. Executive Director's Corner. 2021

[44] United Nations Economic and Social Commission for Asia and the Pacific. Reducing Vulnerability and Exposure to Disasters: The Asia-Pacific Disaster Report 2012. Bangkok, Thailand: United Nations; 2012

[45] Unisdr W. Disaster Risk and Resilience. Thematic Think Piece, UN System Task Force on the Post-2015 UN Development Agenda. Geneva, Switzerland: UN; 2012

[46] Peduzzi P, Chatenoux B, Dao H, De Bono A, Deichmann U, Giuliani G, et al. The Global Risk Analysis for the 2009 Global Assessment Report on Disaster Risk Reduction. Davos: International Disaster and Risk Conference (IDRC); 2010

[47] Piepiora Z, Belarga O, Alindogan MA, Arcos VHR. The

Philippine disaster management system during large scale disasters. International Multidisciplinary Scientific GeoConference: SGEM. 2016;**3**:187-194

[48] Chersan I-C. Corporate responsibility reporting according to global reporting initiative: An international comparison. The Audit Financiar Journal. 2016;**14**(136):424-435

[49] Selby D, Kagawa F. Disaster Risk Reduction in School Curricula: Case Studies from Thirty Countries. Switzerland/France: UNESCO/UNICEF; 2012

[50] Rajesh G, Chhabra KG, Shetty PJ, Prasad KV, Javali SB. A survey on disaster management among postgraduate students in a private dental institution in India. American Journal of Disaster Medicine. 2011;**6**(5):309-318

[51] Kobashi Y, Shimazu Y, Sonoda Y, Saito H, Yoshida M, Tsubokura M. Maturing of public-private-people partnership (4P): Lessons from 4P for triple disaster and subsequently COVID-19 pandemic in Fukushima. Journal of Global Health. 2022;**12**:03028

[52] Minato Disaster Medical Care System Study G. Bottom-up approach to establish coordination mechanisms for disaster preparedness among largely private health-care providers in Central Tokyo. Disaster Medicine and Public Health Preparedness. 2021;**17**:e64

[53] Ikeda M, Palakhamarn T. Economic Damage from Natural Hazards and Local Disaster Management Plans in Japan and Thailand. Jakarta, Indonesia: Economic Research Institute for ASEAN and East Asia; 2020

[54] Golikova T. About the measures aimed to improve labor conditions, preserve employees life and health. In: Report Made at the Meeting of the Russian Government on October 27, 2011. Vol. 1. Russia: Health and Safety and Accidents Prevention in Construction Industry; 2012. pp. 7-11

Chapter 3

Job Stress and Its Management

Mohammad Bagher Hasanvand

Abstract

Stress is an unavoidable reality of life originated from various sources, including daily challenges, significant life changes, and workplace pressures. This chapter delves into the nature of stress, particularly focusing on job-related stress, its causes, and its effects on both mental and physical health. Stress is a response to any challenge that disrupts the body's equilibrium, whether due to external or internal factors. The chapter categorizes stress into several types, including acute, chronic, episodic acute, post-traumatic, situational, workplace, and social stress, each with distinct triggers and impacts on mental and physical health. Job stress is highlighted as a significant type of stress, caused by factors such as excessive workload, conflicts with colleagues, and job insecurity. The objectives of this chapter aimed at reducing impact of stress are: increasing awareness, behavioral changes, stress management skills, problem-solving skills, support networks, time management. Understanding the different types of stress and their symptoms, from physical manifestations such as headaches and fatigue to emotional responses like anxiety and depression, is crucial. Ultimately, the chapter advocates for a proactive approach to managing job stress, emphasizing that while stress cannot be entirely eliminated, its detrimental effects can be reduced through awareness, behavioral adjustments, and effective stress management practices.

Keywords: stress, job stress, stress management skills, mental health, reducing stress

1. Introduction

Despite considerable research on stress and anxiety and seemingly countless approaches to managing and reducing stress, stress is an unavoidable fact of life. We all live with uncertainties, problems, illness, aging, death, and the inability to fully control the events of life. Stress is defined as any challenge to the body's equilibrium (also known as homeostasis). These challenges can range from minor inconveniences like weather changes to major stressors like distressing global news, approaching deadlines, environmental pollution, catching a cold, fluctuating blood pressure, hunger pangs, fatigue, inflammation, sleep deprivation, consuming processed foods, or emotional distress. Stress can manifest in various forms, from real, life-threatening challenges to hidden stressors like worry, feelings of inadequacy, or a defective immune system that cannot mount a strong antibody response. For the brain, anything that challenges the body's homeostasis qualifies as stress, whether physical, psychological, emotional, real, or imagined. Until the brain perceives that your state of equilibrium is challenged, it counts as stress, and with it, a physiological stress response is always triggered to resolve the problem so that you can adapt and ultimately survive.

Achieving total elimination of stress is neither practical nor advisable. Instead, the focus should be on removing unnecessary stressors and effectively managing the unavoidable ones. Although common sources of stress are widely recognized, individual responses to stress can differ significantly. Stress can originate from various sources, known as stressors. Since our perception of what is "stressful" is shaped by our unique interpretations of life events—based on a combination of personality traits, available resources, and habitual thought patterns—a situation perceived as "stressful" by one person may be seen as merely "challenging" by another. In simple terms, what is a stressor for an individual may not be perceived as stressful by another. While individual stressors may vary, certain situations tend to be more universally stressful and can increase the risk of burnout.

For instance, when we find ourselves in situations where there are many demands on us, but we have little control and few choices, we are likely to experience stress. Additionally, we may feel stressed when we are not well-prepared, in situations where we might be heavily judged by others, or where the consequences of failure are severe or unpredictable. Many people experience stress due to their jobs, relationships, financial issues, and health problems, as well as more trivial things like clutter or busy schedules. Learning coping skills for these stressors can help reduce your experience of stress. Stress is a natural reaction of the body to stressful and threatening situations. There are different types of stress, including:

Acute stress: This type of stress is in response to a temporary stressful situation, such as an exam, debate, or short-term deadline. If not managed, it can harm a person's health [1, 2].

Chronic stress: This type of stress continues for long periods of time and may result from a persistent stressful situation, such as an unhappy marriage, financial or work problems. Chronic stress can lead to chronic diseases [1].

Explosive stress (episodic acute stress): This type of stress consists of a combination of acute and chronic stress and is more common in people who live an exciting and active life. These people may regularly face stressful situations [1].

Post-traumatic stress: This type of stress occurs after experiencing an accident or threatening event, such as war, rape, or natural disasters. People may suffer from symptoms such as nightmares, flashbacks, and chronic anxiety [3, 4].

Situational stress: This type of stress is related to specific circumstances and events, such as marriage, divorce, job change, or moving to a new city. This stress usually subsides as the specific situation resolves [3].

Workplace stress: This type of stress is caused by factors in the work environment, such as work pressure, problems with colleagues, job insecurity, and a mismatch between expectations and performance [5].

Social stress: This type of stress comes from social interactions, such as fear of being judged, worry about being accepted by others, and social anxiety.

Each type of stress can have specific symptoms and effects, including psychological, physiological, and emotional effects. The importance of recognizing and managing stress is very important in improving personal and social health [5, 6]. Stress means different things to different people in different situations. A practical definition of stress, which is compatible with many human situations, is a condition in which a person becomes agitated and distressed by an uncontrollable unpleasant challenge. For example, getting stuck in heavy traffic on the highway, being a belligerent employer, having unpaid bills, or encountering a predatory animal [7, 8].

Stress can be defined as any change that induces physical, emotional, or psychological strain. It is your body's response to anything that requires attention or action. Everyone experiences stress to some degree, as the human body is designed to experience and respond to stress. When you encounter changes or challenges (stressors), your body produces physical and psychological responses to help you adapt to new circumstances [7].

Stress can be positive, keeping us alert, motivated, and prepared to avoid danger. For example, if you have an important exam coming up, your stress response may help your body work harder and stay more focused. However, prolonged or excessive stress without periods of relaxation can be detrimental to our well-being. How we react to stress significantly impacts our overall health. Sometimes, addressing the source of stress is the solution. Other times, changing our perspective or coping mechanisms can be more effective. Depending on the circumstances, the stress response can lead to a fight-or-flight reaction. The magnitude of stress and its physiological consequences are influenced by your perception of your ability to cope with the stressor [8].

The intensity of the stress response and its physical effects depend on how capable we feel in managing the situation. Therefore, understanding the relationship between stress, physical health, and mental health is crucial for overall well-being.

2. Objectives of this chapter

The main objectives of the chapter on stress and its management are to provide effective ways to reduce the negative impacts of stress on individuals' mood and performance. Some of the behavioral goals in this process include:

1. *Awareness*: Increasing awareness about the causes and factors leading to stress, its effects on the body and mind, and methods to reduce it.

2. *Change in undesirable behaviors*: Identifying unhealthy or inappropriate behavioral patterns that can increase stress and striving to change them positively.

3. *Enhancement of stress management skills*: Teaching various methods such as breathing techniques, relaxation, meditation, and exercise to help reduce stress levels.

4. *Improvement of problem-solving skills*: Educating effective methods to cope with problems and handle stressful situations so that individuals can deal with them better.

5. *Strengthening the support network*: Creating and reinforcing social relationships and support networks in the workplace or personal life, which can help reduce feelings of loneliness and increase human support.

6. *Time management*: Teaching time management skills and appropriate planning to reduce pressures and stress related to time constraints.

3. Fear vs. anxiety: Understanding distinguishes

Stress is closely linked to fear and anxiety. The definitions of fear and anxiety vary greatly and depend to some extent on subjective assessment. However, Craske et al., in their seminal review "What is an Anxiety Disorder?", use Barlow's concepts to state: "*anxiety is a future-oriented mood state associated with preparation for possible, upcoming negative events; and fear is an alarm response to present or imminent danger (real or perceived). This view of human fear and anxiety is comparable to the animal predatory imminence continuum. That is, anxiety corresponds to an animal's state during a potential predatory attack and fear corresponds to an animal's state during predator contact or imminent contact*" [1, 9, 10].

4. What happens to the body during stress?

Stress leads to feelings of fear and anxiety. The body's autonomic nervous system controls heart rate, breathing, changes in vision, and more. The body's response to stress is often termed the "fight-or-flight" response, a mechanism designed to help us manage challenging situations. However, prolonged or chronic stress can weaken the body's defenses, leading to a range of physical, emotional, and behavioral issues. Physical symptoms of stress include:

- Bodily aches and pains
- A pain in the chest or a racing heart
- Fatigue or having difficulty sleeping
- Headache, confusion or tremors
- Elevated blood pressure
- Muscle tightness, especially in the neck and shoulders
- Grinding the teeth and clenching the jaw
- Stomach or digestive problems
- Decreased libido and difficulty in sex
- Weak immune system
- Stress can lead to emotional and psychological symptoms such as:
- Change in mood
- Low energy
- Anxiety or irritability
- Depression

- Panic attack
- Sadness

5. Common signs and symptoms of excessive stress

Stress is an inevitable part of life that affects everyone, arising from various pressures such as work, relationships, and financial challenges. Whether you are facing everyday stress, long-term chronic stress, or significant life challenges like illness or divorce, the impact of stress can be substantial, affecting both your physical and mental well-being. How can you determine if the level of stress you are experiencing is detrimental to your health?

This question can be challenging to answer due to several factors:

- *Variety of effects*: Stress manifests in numerous ways. While some signs are apparent, others may not be noticeable until they become severe.
- *Individual differences*: People experience and react to stress differently; some are more affected than others, and the manifestations can vary widely.
- *Symptom confusion*: Stress can mimic the symptoms of other illnesses, partly because it lowers immunity, making one more susceptible to various health issues. This can lead to confusion between stress symptoms and those of other conditions.
- *Adaptation to stress*: Individuals who have grown up in stressful environments might perceive stress as their normal state, making it harder to identify stress symptoms until their stress levels decrease significantly.

6. Common symptoms that indicate you are under a lot of stress

While the impact of stress varies from person to person, certain signs are commonly associated with elevated stress levels. If you are experiencing any of the following, it might indicate you are under significant stress: [10–12].

6.1 Headaches

Some types of headaches can be triggered by stress. In tension headaches, it feels like you have a band wrapped around your head and the band is slowly tightening. If you are experiencing more headaches, especially tension headaches, stress could be to blame.

6.2 Frequent colds or flu

There is an inverse relationship between stress and immunity, meaning that the higher your stress level, the less effective your immune system is in general. This is true for stressors that are more intense or stressors that are more chronic. A weakened immune system increases vulnerability to a range of illnesses, from common colds to more severe health problems. Consequently, individuals experiencing high levels of stress may find themselves falling ill more frequently.

6.3 Sleep problems

There are many ways that stress affects sleep. Stress can make it harder to fall asleep and cause you to wake up during the night. A lot of stress can rob you of sleep, and your body can repair itself less during the sleep process [13].

6.4 General anxiety

Anxiety is a natural human emotion that can be beneficial in certain situations. However, when anxiety becomes persistent, excessive, and interferes with daily life, it may indicate underlying stress or a more serious mental health condition like generalized anxiety disorder. If you are struggling with persistent anxiety, seeking professional help from a mental health professional is recommended.

6.5 Vague thinking

In response to stress, your body releases hormones that allow you to quickly fight or flee. However, it is designed for rare and short-lived stresses. When this stress response is overstimulated, it can actually make you think less quickly.

7. How is stress diagnosed?

Stress is a subjective phenomenon and cannot be measured by experiments. Only the person experiencing it can determine if it exists or what it feels like. A health care provider may use a questionnaire to understand your stress and how it affects your life. If you have chronic stress, your doctor can evaluate for stress-related symptoms. For example, high blood pressure can be diagnosed and treated.

7.1 The major causes of stress

Stress is a universal human experience, yet its triggers vary widely from person to person. While stress is a normal part of life, its impact differs individually. For instance, a traffic jam might infuriate one person but merely annoy another. Similarly, a disagreement with a friend can be a significant upset for some, while others may quickly move on. Below are the factors that lead to stress: [14–16].

7.2 Financial concerns

Financial concerns are a primary stressor for Americans. According to the American Psychological Association (APA), money consistently tops the list of stress triggers. A 2015 APA survey revealed that a substantial majority of Americans experienced money-related stress within the past month, with many citing it as a significant source of worry.

Symptoms of financial stress may include:

- Arguing with loved ones about money
- Fear of opening messages or answering the phone

- Feeling guilty about spending money on unnecessary things
- Anxiety and feeling worried about money

Prolonged financial stress can have severe consequences for overall health. It can manifest physically as elevated blood pressure, persistent headaches, digestive issues, chest pain, sleep disturbances, and a general sense of unwellness. Moreover, financial stress is linked to a range of chronic health conditions including depression, anxiety, skin problems, diabetes, and arthritis.

7.3 Job

According to the Centers for Disease Control and Prevention, Compared to two decades ago, Americans are putting in eight percent more hours on the job, and 13 percent are holding down second jobs. These extended work hours are taking a toll, with at least 40 percent of workers reporting job-related stress and a quarter feeling burned out. Things like overwork, lack of job security, job dissatisfaction and conflicts with the boss and/or colleagues can lead to job stress. Whether you are worried about a particular project, feel like you have been treated unfairly, or prioritize your career over everything else, it can affect many aspects of your life, including personal relationships and mental and physical health. Factors outside the job, such as a person's mental state, general health, personal life, and the level of emotional support outside of work also play a role in job stress [14].

Symptoms of work-related stress can be physical and psychological, including: [17–19].

- Anxiety
- Depression
- Difficulty concentrating or making decisions
- Fatigue
- Headache
- Heart beat
- Mood swings
- Muscle tension and pain
- Stomach problems

Some people may feel a lot of pressure and have trouble coping, which can also affect their behavior. Job stress may force people to: [11, 17].

- Reduction of creativity and initiative
- Disinterest

- Decrease performance
- Increase in sick days
- Isolation and seclusion
- Low levels of patience and increased levels of frustration
- Personal relationship problems

7.4 Personal relationships

In our whole life there are people who cause us stress. Toxic individuals can infiltrate any aspect of our lives, from family and friendship to romantic partnerships and professional settings. These harmful relationships can significantly impact both our physical and mental well-being. Romantic relationships are particularly susceptible to stress, and persistent strain can jeopardize the bond between partners. Common stressful factors in relationships are:

- Being too busy to spend time with each other and share responsibilities
- Lack of intimacy and sex due to busyness, health problems, and other reasons
- Existence of abuse or control in the relationship
- Alcohol or drug use in person and/or partner
- Thinking of separation and divorce in the person or his wife

You may also be avoiding or fighting with the person, or easily irritated by their presence. Stress arising from personal relationships often mirrors the symptoms of general stress, encompassing physical ailments, sleep disturbances, depression, and anxiety. It's important to recognize that even our online interactions, through platforms like Facebook and Instagram, can contribute to this stress. For example, in social networks, the tendency to compare oneself with others naturally increases, which can lead to stress caused by feelings of inadequacy [20].

7.5 Parenting as a source of stress

The demands of modern parenthood, including balancing employment, household responsibilities, and childcare, often lead to elevated stress levels. Chronic parental stress can manifest in negative parenting behaviors such as harshness, criticism, and authoritarianism. Furthermore, it can erode the quality of parent-child relationships, hindering open communication and fostering conflict. Factors contributing to parental stress include financial strain, long work hours, single parenthood, marital discord, and raising children with special needs. Parents of children with developmental or behavioral disorders are particularly susceptible to heightened stress. Research consistently indicates that parents of children with autism experience significantly higher levels of stress compared to parents of neurotypical children [11, 21, 22].

7.6 Busy and everyday life

Everyday hassles can contribute significantly to overall stress levels. Minor inconveniences such as lost keys or forgotten items may seem insignificant, but their cumulative impact can lead to anxiety and negatively affect physical and mental well-being. The relentless pace of modern life has exacerbated stress levels. People are busier than ever before, juggling multiple responsibilities. While some have no choice but to work long hours, others find it difficult to decline additional commitments due to a sense of obligation. This overextension often comes at the expense of self-care, as individuals struggle to prioritize basic needs like nutrition and exercise [21, 23].

7.7 Personality and stress

Individual personality traits significantly influence stress levels. While personality is shaped by various factors, it can also independently contribute to stress. For instance, extroverted individuals often report lower stress levels and benefit from stronger social support networks, acting as a buffer against stress. Conversely, perfectionists may impose unnecessary pressure on themselves due to their high standards, leading to heightened emotional and physical strain. This tendency can also create stress for those around them.

Now, one of the types of stress that increases day by day due to the complexities of societies and shows its effects in the lives of people is occupational stress, which we will discuss more about in the rest of the chapter [10, 24].

8. Occupational stress: What is occupational stress?

Job stress is an emotional response that occurs when faced with uncontrollable, unpredictable job situations or in situations where there is excessive work pressure. This stress affects people in different ways. In cases where there is a lot of work stress on a person, very minor and small things (such as the failure of the copier when you need it) can also cause strong reactions from people.

Occupational stress has different symptoms. These symptoms are classified into two general categories: [12, 24].

- Physical symptoms
- Psychological symptoms

Physical symptoms caused by job stress include:

He mentioned headache, sleep disturbance, digestive problems, problems in concentration, chronic fatigue, pain in muscles and tendons, undereating or overeating an d chronic diseases. Psychological symptoms caused by job stress include: Anxiety, irritability, anger, job dissatisfaction, demoralization and family problems such as marital conflicts or problems in parenting.

8.1 Occupational stress factors

8.1.1 Individual factors

Some personality traits make people experience more job stress than others. For example, people who always suffer from anxiety and worry (pervasive anxiety) in the workplace are also more stressed when faced with job duties. Or that the person does not have time management and planning skills and as a result cannot handle assigned tasks well. Also, the lack of appropriateness of personality traits and capabilities required in a specific job can also lead to job stress [19, 25].

Perfectionism is also one of the effective factors in job stress. There are two forms of perfectionism, negative and positive. Positive perfectionism can encourage people to constantly seek their own growth and development and take steps toward personal development. But negative perfectionism is a big obstacle to people's growth and development. People with negative perfectionism experience a lot of job stress. Because they are afraid of making mistakes, they are constantly worried about doing something wrong, and they cannot tolerate the slightest criticism, and if they make a mistake, they constantly review this incident in their minds and suffer from rumination. The set of these factors causes the job satisfaction of perfectionist (negative) people to decrease and experience a lot of stress and anxiety [11, 25].

8.1.2 Organizational factors

8.1.2.1 Excessive work pressure

One of the most common causes of occupational stress is exposure to environments that put a lot of pressure on people. Employees in such environments are always faced with a lot of accumulated work, which causes them to experience a lot of stress.

8.1.2.2 The unpredictability of the work environment

Working in environments where people's duties are not defined properly and at any moment a person may face an unexpected situation causes a lot of job stress to people.

8.1.2.3 Competitive environment

If people are working in an environment where there is no friendly atmosphere between employees and people are constantly competing with each other, an atmosphere full of stress and anxiety is created [20, 25].

8.1.3 Stress and work performance

Anxiety and stress are not negative phenomena by themselves. Studies have shown that stress can sometimes be positive. Job stress helps us to be more alert and perform better in some situations. But stress can only be beneficial when experienced in the short term. Prolonged or excessive stress can seriously disrupt our physical and mental performance. One of the negative effects of job stress is a drop in work performance. When people are under tension and stress, certain hormones called adrenaline and noradrenaline are released in their body. These hormones lead to increased heart rate and blood pressure. These hormones can also reduce blood flow to the surface of the skin and lead to reduced digestive activity. Cortisol is another hormone that is released in response to stress and increases energy. As a result of these changes, people under job stress may feel headache, muscle tension, pain, nausea, indigestion and dizziness. All these changes are the body's mechanism to deal with stress and pressure; But if they continue continuously and the level of anxiety does not return to the basic state, the level of these hormones remains high and as a result, the normal functioning of the body is disturbed. When people do not feel well physically and are constantly involved in medical problems, naturally they cannot perform successfully and they will have low concentration in doing things [23, 26].

8.2 Occupational stress management

The role and importance of human resources today is not hidden from managers. Many HR managers are very careful in selecting their employees and try to select talented people. Paying attention to the suitability of personality traits and job duties is very important; But the work does not end there. Human resource managers should also pay attention to the personal growth and development of their employees. Job stress management is very important in increasing the work quality and job productivity of people, and if employees can control their job stress well, they will be able to handle their job duties and will have effective and useful communication with other colleagues. Job stress management is effective in reducing anger in interpersonal relationships and prevents employee burnout [19, 26].

Regardless of your occupation, you can implement strategies to shield yourself from the detrimental impacts of stress, enhance job satisfaction, and improve overall well-being. A certain level of stress can actually be beneficial, boosting focus, energy, and the ability to conquer new challenges. However, in today's fast-paced environment, the workplace can often feel like an emotional whirlwind. Prolonged exposure to demanding workloads, tight deadlines, and escalating expectations can lead to feelings of anxiety, exhaustion, and overwhelm. When stress becomes overwhelming, it negatively affects both physical and mental health, as well as job performance.

While you cannot control every aspect of your work environment, you do possess the power to take action. If job stress is adversely affecting your work, health, or personal life, it's time to make changes. No matter your career path or the level of stress you encounter, there are numerous techniques to reduce stress and regain a sense of control within your job.

Common Workplace Stressors Include:

- Fear of job loss
- Increased overtime due to staff reductions
- Pressure to excel without commensurate rewards
- Constant pressure to perform at peak levels
- Limited autonomy in work processes

8.3 Warning signs of workplace stress

Feeling overwhelmed at work can erode confidence and lead to irritability, anger, or social withdrawal. Other indicators of excessive job-related stress include:

- Emotional turmoil such as anxiety, irritability, or depression
- Loss of interest or motivation in work

- Sleep disturbances and persistent fatigue
- Difficulty concentrating and maintaining focus
- Physical symptoms like muscle tension, headaches, or stomach issues
- Reduced social interaction and isolation
- Changes in sexual desire
- Reliance on alcohol or drugs as a coping mechanism

8.3.1 Tip 1: Connect and conquer stress

Sharing your burdens with others can significantly alleviate stress. Talking openly about your challenges and receiving support can provide immense relief. Remember, your confidant does not need to solve your problems; their empathetic listening is invaluable.

Cultivate strong relationships with colleagues. A supportive work environment can act as a buffer against stress. Reciprocity is key; be there for your colleagues as well. If you lack close work friendships, initiate social interactions during breaks.

Prioritize connections with friends and family. A strong support network is essential for overall well-being. Isolation can exacerbate stress, so nurture your relationships. Expand your social circle by joining clubs or volunteering. Helping others can be incredibly rewarding and provide a much-needed distraction from personal stress. Remember, building and maintaining social connections is an investment in your mental health.

8.3.2 Tip 2: Feed your body, enhance your mind

When work demands dominate, physical health often takes a backseat. However, a strong body supports a resilient mind. Simple steps can boost energy, mood, and overall well-being.

Regular exercise is a powerful tool for stress management. Aim for at least 30 minutes of moderate-intensity activity most days. Activities like walking, running, or dancing can be particularly beneficial. When stress levels rise, short breaks for physical movement can help regain composure. Nutrition plays a crucial role in managing stress. Consuming balanced meals throughout the day helps stabilize energy levels and mood. Limit sugary and processed foods, as they can exacerbate stress symptoms. Incorporate foods rich in omega-3 fatty acids, such as fatty fish and flaxseed, for their mood-boosting properties. Avoid excessive caffeine, nicotine, and alcohol, as they can contribute to anxiety and disrupt sleep. Remember, small changes in diet and exercise can have a significant impact on your overall health and ability to cope with stress.

8.3.3 Tip 3: Prioritize sleep for optimal performance

Insufficient sleep can significantly hinder daytime productivity, creativity, and problem-solving abilities. Adequate rest is essential for effectively managing job responsibilities and coping with workplace stress.

Establish consistent sleep and wake times, even on weekends. Maintain a balanced diet and create a soothing sleep environment. Aim for 7 to 9 hours of uninterrupted sleep each night. Invest in a comfortable sleep setup, including mattress, pillows, and bedding. Sleep patterns. Instead, engage in calming activities like reading or listening to gentle music. Shift work can disrupt sleep patterns and increase stress. Gradually adjust your sleep-wake cycle by exposure to bright light upon waking and using blackout curtains during daytime sleep. Limit consecutive night shifts and avoid frequent shift rotations. Create a dark, quiet sleep environment during the day. By prioritizing sleep, you can enhance overall well-being, improve job performance, and better manage stress.

8.3.4 Tip 4: Master time and tasks

When job pressures become overwhelming, simple strategies can restore balance and control.

8.4 Manage your time effectively

- *Prioritize well-being*: Balance work with personal life, social connections, and rest to prevent burnout.

- *Start stress-free*: Begin your day calmly by allowing extra time for your morning routine.

- *Recharge regularly*: Take short breaks throughout the day to rest and refocus. Step away from work during lunch to improve productivity.

- *Set healthy boundaries*: Establish clear work-life separations to avoid constant work-related demands.

- *Avoid overextension*: Focus on essential tasks and decline additional commitments when necessary.

8.5 Organize your workload

- *Tackle important tasks first*: Prioritize and complete high-priority items to reduce stress.

- *Break down large projects*: Divide complex tasks into smaller, manageable steps.

- *Share the load*: Delegate responsibilities to reduce workload and stress.

- *Find common ground*: Collaborate with colleagues to find mutually agreeable solutions and reduce stress.

8.5.1 Tip 5: Overcome stress-inducing habits

Negative thoughts and behaviors can significantly amplify workplace stress. By modifying these habits, you can better manage stress caused by external factors.

- *Embrace imperfection*: Setting unrealistic goals can lead to unnecessary pressure. Celebrate achievements and understand that perfection is unattainable.

- *Cultivate a positive mindset*: Negative thinking drains energy and motivation. Focus on positive aspects of your work, limit exposure to negativity, and recognize small victories.

- *Focus on what you can control*: Many workplace challenges are beyond our influence. Instead of dwelling on uncontrollable factors, concentrate on your responses and actions.

- *Harness the power of humor*: Laughter can be a potent stress reliever. Share jokes or lighthearted moments to improve workplace morale.

- *Create an organized workspace*: A cluttered environment can contribute to stress. Declutter and organize your workspace to enhance efficiency and reduce frustration.

8.6 Be proactive in your job responsibilities

Feelings of uncertainty, helplessness, or lack of control often contribute to heightened stress levels. To regain a sense of control over your career, consider the following strategies:

- *Communicate with your employer*: Openly discuss workplace stressors with your employer. A productive and happy workforce is beneficial for the company. Instead of general complaints, focus on specific factors impacting your performance.

- *Clarify your role*: Request an updated job description from your supervisor. This can help identify tasks outside your responsibilities and potentially reduce workload.

- *Explore new opportunities*: Consider a transfer within the company to escape a challenging work environment or seek new challenges by taking on different tasks or projects.

- *Prioritize Self-Care*: If burnout is imminent, take a break. A vacation or extended time off can help recharge and provide perspective.

8.7 Seek purpose and satisfaction in your work

Job dissatisfaction and boredom can significantly impact both physical and mental well-being. While a fulfilling dream job may seem unattainable for many, it's possible to find purpose and joy even in less-than-ideal work situations. By focusing on how your contributions benefit others or the value you provide, you can shift your perspective. Cultivating positive relationships with coworkers and identifying enjoyable aspects of your job can also contribute to a more fulfilling work experience. A change in attitude can empower you to regain a sense of control and purpose.

8.8 What strategies can managers or employers use to alleviate workplace stress?

Work-related stress can significantly impact employees, leading to decreased productivity, absenteeism, and higher turnover rates. As managers and supervisors, you can play a crucial role in mitigating workplace stress. A fundamental step is to serve as a positive example. By maintaining composure under pressure, you can inspire your team to do the same.

Engage in open dialog with your employees. Discuss specific factors contributing to job-related stress. Address easily resolvable issues such as equipment malfunctions, staffing shortages, or inadequate supervisor feedback. Sharing information openly can alleviate employee uncertainty about their roles and future within the company. Prioritize one-on-one conversations with employees to actively listen to their concerns. This demonstrates care and understanding, which can alleviate stress for both parties, even when immediate solutions are unavailable.

Empower employees by involving them in decisions that impact their work. For instance, seek employee input on workplace policies. This collaborative approach fosters a stronger sense of commitment. Additionally, ensure that workloads are reasonable and deadlines are achievable by carefully considering staff capabilities and resources.

Specify your Clear Expectations. Clearly define employee roles, responsibilities, and goals. Implement fair and consistent management practices that align with organizational values. Give them motivations and rewards to acknowledge employee achievements. Praise work successes verbally and across the organization. Balance high-pressure periods with less demanding tasks. Create opportunities for social interaction among employees to strengthen relationships and reduce stress [27–29].

9. Discussion and conclusion

Stress is a natural physiological response where the body reacts to adverse and stressful conditions. Stress can originate from everyday issues such as heavy traffic, migration, financial problems, or job loss. However, prolonged stress can lead to more serious issues like an increased risk of heart disease, depression, and anxiety. Stress management refers to the set of methods and techniques used to reduce and control stress. These include both physical and psychological methods that help an individual eliminate or cope with stress. Breathing techniques, meditation, yoga, exercise, and promoting happiness are among the methods that can be effective in managing stress. Additionally, creating a regular schedule, increasing recreational activities, and supporting social networks can also improve stress management.

Furthermore, utilizing negotiation strategies, effective planning, and practicing effective communication can also contribute to reducing stress and enhancing stress management. The importance of leveraging supportive situations and avoiding intermediary situations also plays a significant role in stress management. Consequently, stress management is highly important as it can lead to improved quality of life in the long term and prevent the negative effects of stress on physical and mental health. Therefore, it is suggested:

- *Meditatio* – Practice meditation to calm your mind.

- *Exercitia* – Engage in physical exercise; it helps release endorphins.

- *Respiratio profundus* – Take deep breaths to enhance relaxation.
- *Naturae ambulatio* – Take a walk in nature to recharge.
- *Musica auscultatio* – Listen to calming music to soothe your nerves.
- *Socius tempus* – Spend time with friends or loved ones for support.
- *Somnus satis* – Ensure you get enough sleep to recuperate.
- *Cibus sanus* – Eat a healthy diet to maintain your energy levels.
- *Ars creatrix* – Engage in creative activities like drawing or writing.
- *Temporalitas* – Allocate time for yourself and practice self-care.

Author details

Mohammad Bagher Hasanvand
Department of Psychology and Education of Exceptional Children, Faculty of Psychology and Educational Sciences, Allameh Tabataba'I University, Tehran, Iran

*Address all correspondence to: b.hasanvand06@gmail.com

References

[1] Craske MG, Rauch SL, Ursano R, Prenoveau J, Pine DS, Zinbarg RE. What is an anxiety disorder? Depression and Anxiety. 2009;**26**:1066-1085

[2] Stress, Social Support, and the Buffering Hypothesis. – PsycNET. Available from: https://doi.apa.org/doiLanding?doi=10.1037%2F0033-2909.98.2.310 [Accessed: November 15, 2021]

[3] Rozental JM. Tension-type headache, chronic tension-type headache, and other chronic headache types. In: Benzon HT, Raja SN, Liu SS, Fishman SM, Cohen SP, editors. Essentials of Pain Medicine. 4th ed. Philadelphia, PA: Elsevier; 2018: chap 20

[4] Toussaint L, Nguyen QA, Roettger C, Dixon K, Offenbächer M, Kohls N, et al. Effectiveness of progressive muscle relaxation, deep breathing, and guided imagery in promoting psychological and physiological states of relaxation. Evidence-based Complementary and Alternative Medicine. 2021;**2021**:e5924040. DOI: 10.1155/2021/5924040

[5] Cohen S, Janicki-Deverts D, Doyle WJ, et al. Chronic stress, glucocorticoid receptor resistance, inflammation, and disease risk. Proceedings of the National Academy of Sciences of the United States of America. 2012;**109**(16):5995-5999

[6] McEwen BS. Stress, adaptation, and disease: Allostasis and allostatic load. Annals of the New York Academy of Sciences. 1998;**840**:33-44. DOI: 10.1111/j.1749-6632.1998.tb09546.x

[7] National Institute of Mental Health. Generalized Anxiety Disorder: When Worry Gets out of Control. NIHM; 2016. Available from: https://www.nimh.nih.gov/health/publications/generalized-anxiety-disorder-gad

[8] Estes A, Olson E, Sullivan K, et al. Parenting-related stress and psychological distress in mothers of toddlers with autism spectrum disorders. Brain & Development. 2013;**35**(2):133-138

[9] Can YS, Iles-Smith H, Chalabianloo N, Ekiz D, Fernández-Álvarez J, Repetto C, et al. How to relax in stressful situations: A smart stress reduction system. Healthcare. 2020;**8**(2):100. DOI: 10.3390/healthcare8020100

[10] Saleh D, Camart N, Sbeira F, Romo L. Can we learn to manage stress? A randomized controlled trial carried out on university students. PLoS One. 2018;**13**(9):e0200997. DOI: 10.1371/journal.pone.0200997

[11] Rongjun Y. Stress potentiates decision biases: A stress induced deliberation-to-intuition (SIDI) model. Neurobiology of Stress. 2016;**3**:83-95

[12] Yang CC, Barrós-Loscertales A, Li M, et al. Alterations in brain structure and amplitude of low-frequency after 8 weeks of mindfulness meditation training in meditation-naïve subjects. Scientific Reports. 2019;**9**(1):10977. DOI: 10.1038/s41598-019-47470-4

[13] Choi DW, Chun SY, Lee SA, Han KT, Park EC. Association between sleep duration and perceived stress: Salaried worker in circumstances of high workload. International Journal of Environmental Research and Public Health. 2018;**15**(4):796. DOI: 10.3390/ijerph15040796

[14] American Psychological Association. Stress in America: Paying with our Health. American Psychological Association; 2015. Retrieved from: https://www.apa.org/news/press/releases/stress/2015/stress-report.pdf

[15] Wunsch K, Wurst R, Von dawans B, Strahler J, Kasten N, Fuchs R. Habitual and acute exercise effects on salivary biomarkers in response to psychosocial stress. Psychoneuroendocrinology. 2019;**106**:216-225. DOI: 10.1016/j.psyneuen.2019.03.015

[16] Yaribeygi H, Panahi Y, Sahraei H, Johnston TP, Sahebkar A. The impact of stress on body function: A review. EXCLI Journal. 2017;**16**:1057-1072

[17] Centers for Disease Control and Prevention (CDC). Stress...at Work. Centers for Disease Control and Prevention (CDC); 2014. Retrieved from: https://www.cdc.gov/niosh/docs/2014-134/pdfs/2014-134.pdf

[18] Cohen S, Janicki-Deverts D, Miller GE. Psychological stress and disease. JAMA. 2007;**298**(14):1685-1687. DOI: 10.1001/jama.298.14.1685

[19] Chrousos GP. Stress and disorders of the stress system. Nature Reviews Endocrinology. 2009;**5**(8):468-475. DOI: 10.1038/nrendo.2009.152

[20] Kemeny ME. The psychobiology of stress. Current Directions in Psychological Science. 2003;**12**(4):124-129. DOI: 10.1111/1467-8721.01247

[21] Cleveland Clinic. Stress. Cleveland Clinic; 2015. Retrieved from: https://my.clevelandclinic.org/health/diseases/9431-stress

[22] Thoits PA. Stress and health: Concepts and sociological approaches. Journal of Health and Social Behavior. 2010;**51**(S):S41-S53. DOI: 10.1177/0022146510383499

[23] Bhui K, Dinos S, Galant-Miecznikowska M, de Jongh B, Stansfeld S. Perceptions of work stress causes and effective interventions in employees working in public, private and non-governmental organisations: A qualitative study. BJPsych Bulletin. 2016;**40**(6):318-325. DOI: 10.1192/pb.bp.115.050823

[24] Tsai YC, Liu CH. Factors and symptoms associated with work stress and health-promoting lifestyles among hospital staff: A pilot study in Taiwan. BMC Health Services Research. 2012;**12**:199

[25] Falconier MK, Nussbeck F, Bodenmann G, Schneider H, Bradbury T. Stress from daily hassles in couples: Its effects on intradyadic stress, relationship satisfaction, and physical and psychological well-being. Journal of Marital and Family Therapy. 2015;**41**(2):221-235

[26] Rus HM, Tiemensma J. Social media under the skin: Facebook use after acute stress impairs cortisol recovery. Frontiers in Psychology. 2017;**8**:1609

[27] Maulik PK. Workplace stress: A neglected aspect of mental health wellbeing. The Indian Journal of Medical Research. 2017;**146**(4):441-444. Available from: https://www.ncbi.nlm.nih.gov/pmc/articles/PMC5819024/

[28] Penedo FJ, Dahn JR. Exercise and well-being: A review of mental and physical health benefits associated with physical activity. Current Directions in Psychological Science. 2005;**14**(5):199-203. DOI: 10.1111/j.0963-7214.2005.00357.x

[29] Wang W, Sakata K, Komiya A, Li Y. What makes employees' work so stressful? Effects of vertical leadership and horizontal management on employees' stress. Frontiers in Psychology. 2020;**11**:340. DOI: 10.3389/fpsyg.2020.00340

Chapter 4

Ergonomic Interventions in Risk Reduction

Ehsan Garosi, Fatemeh Sheikh and Mahsa Goodarzi

Abstract

Ergonomics is a dynamic and multidisciplinary field that explores the interactions between people and various elements within systems. Its primary goal is to optimize health, performance, productivity, and satisfaction through the design and implementation of targeted interventions. These systems can range from simple setups, such as pen-and-paper, to complex sociotechnical infrastructures like large factories or agricultural systems. While its applications span all human activities, ergonomics often centers on workplace laws and occupational knowledge. This chapter highlights the significant role of ergonomic interventions in reducing workplace risks, particularly musculoskeletal disorders (MSDs). Modern ergonomic approaches leveraging wearable technology, virtual reality (VR), and the Internet of Things (IoT) offer innovative solutions that support both physical and cognitive aspects of ergonomics. By focusing on adaptable and data-driven interventions, future ergonomic practices can align more closely with evolving workplace needs, enhancing risk management outcomes and improving employee well-being and productivity. Moreover, ergonomics impacts not only computer systems but also mobile platforms, wearable technology, IoT devices, and Artificial Intelligence (AI)-driven applications. With the integration of machine learning and other emerging technologies, ergonomics now extends into real-time monitoring and predictive analytics. This allows for proactive intervention in diverse environments, thereby enhancing both individual well-being and system performance. Our chapter's suggestions are intended for occupational safety specialists and safety managers, highlighting the necessity of continuous efforts and innovative solutions to advance ergonomic practices further.

Keywords: ergonomics, ergonomic intervention, risk reduction, ergonomics risk factors, occupational risk, human factors

1. Introduction

Ergonomics is a relatively new multidisciplinary field of study that examines interactions between people and other system elements. This science addresses the primary objective of the field, which is to optimize health and increase performance, productivity, and satisfaction, through the design and implementation of interventions. According to this concept, a "system" could be either a word written on a paper or the intricate sociotechnical service center structures (such as huge factories or gardens). Ergonomics became recognized as a science in the twentieth century and was taught in psychology and engineering colleges. Ergonomics is a very extensive science that pertains to all human activities, yet it is mostly referred to work law or work knowledge. Using scientific methods to establish ideas, principles, and design tactics, ergonomics has reduced human errors, improved efficacy, increased applicability, and minimized occupational accidents and relative injuries. It also has an impact on computer systems and products. According to the U.S. Bureau of Labor Statistics (BLS), in 2018, there were 900,380 DAFW (days away from work) cases in the U.S. private sector, with 272,780 (or 30%) being cases involving musculoskeletal disorders (MSDs). In 2011, there were 311,840 cases involving MSDs. The incidence rate of cases involving MSDs was 27.2 per 10,000 full-time workers in 2018, and 35.4 in 2011. The median days away from work for cases involving MSDs was 12 in 2018 and it was 11 days in 2011. This information highlights the importance of ergonomics practices and interventions in workplaces.

Impact on risk reduction: The application of ergonomic principles has led to significant reduction in work-related injuries and illnesses, particularly MSDs. Organizations that prioritize ergonomics often report lower injury rates, reduced absenteeism, increased productivity, and improved worker satisfaction. Moreover, the focus on risk reduction in ergonomics has contributed to the development of regulatory standards and guidelines, such as those established by the Occupational Safety and Health Administration (OSHA) and the International Organization for Standardization (ISO), which provide frameworks for implementing ergonomic practices in the workplace.

1.1 Definition and history of ergonomics

The word ergonomics—"the science of work"— is derived from the Greek words "Ergon" (work) and "Nomos" (laws). The fact that the word ergonomics was coined by a Polish scholar, Wojciech Jastrzębowski, in 1857 became widely known when his book in Polish was reprinted with English translation in 1997. The terms ergonomics and human factors are often used interchangeably or as a unit (e.g., human factors/ergonomics—Human Factors Engineering (HFE) or Ergonomics and Human Factors (EHF)), a practice that is adopted by the IEA (International Ergonomics and Human Factors Association). The definition of ergonomics (or human factors) adopted by the IEA in 2000 is the scientific discipline concerned with the understanding of interactions among humans and other elements of a system, and the profession that applies theory, principles, data, and methods to design in order to optimize human well-being and overall system performance.

Early Beginnings: The concept of ergonomics can be traced back to ancient times when humans began designing tools and equipment to enhance their ability to perform tasks. For example, early humans developed tools that were better suited to the hand's natural grip, improving efficiency and reducing strain. However, these early developments were largely intuitive and lacked the systematic approach that characterizes modern ergonomics.

Industrial Revolution: The Industrial Revolution in the eighteenth and nineteenth centuries marked a significant turning point in the development of ergonomics. The rapid mechanization of work processes led to an increase in work-related injuries and health issues, particularly in factory settings. During this time, attention began to shift toward improving working conditions to reduce the physical strain on workers. The introduction of scientific management principles by Frederick Winslow Taylor in the late nineteenth century, which emphasized the optimization of work processes and worker efficiency, laid the groundwork for the formal study of ergonomics.

Twentieth century and the formalization of ergonomics: Ergonomics began to emerge as a distinct field of study in the early twentieth century, particularly during and after World War II. The war effort highlighted the need for improved human-machine interaction, as the design of military equipment and vehicles often led to operator fatigue, errors, and injuries. Researchers began to study human performance and limitations systematically, leading to the development of ergonomic principles that could be applied to improve safety and efficiency. In the 1950s and 1960s, ergonomics gained recognition as a formal discipline, with the establishment of professional organizations such as the Ergonomics Research Society (now the Chartered Institute of Ergonomics and Human Factors) in the United Kingdom (UK). During this period, the focus on risk reduction became more prominent, as researchers and practitioners began to apply ergonomic principles to a wide range of industries, including manufacturing, healthcare, and transportation.

Modern ergonomics: Today, ergonomics is widely recognized as an essential aspect of occupational health and safety. The field has expanded to include various subdisciplines, such as cognitive ergonomics, organizational ergonomics, and physical ergonomics, each focusing on different aspects of human-system interaction. The emphasis on risk reduction in modern ergonomics is evident in the widespread adoption of ergonomic interventions in the workplace. These interventions may include the redesign of workstations to promote neutral postures, the introduction of adjustable furniture and equipment, the implementation of job rotation and micro-breaks to reduce repetitive strain, and the development of training programs to educate workers on safe work practices.

2. Ergonomics domains

Ergonomics is a multidisciplinary field that focuses on optimizing the interaction between humans and their environment to enhance performance, safety, and well-being. It is generally divided into three main domains: *physical ergonomics*, *cognitive ergonomics*, and *organizational ergonomics*. Each of these domains addresses different aspects of human-system interaction.

2.1 Physical ergonomics

Physical ergonomics is concerned with human anatomical, anthropometric, physiological, and biomechanical characteristics as they relate to physical activity. This domain is fundamentally focused on the relationship between the human body and the physical environment, encompassing a wide range of human factors. In addition, it examines how people interact with physical elements, such as tools, equipment, and workspace design. Every section of each domain is explained in the following.

2.1.1 Anthropometry and anatomy

The human body is a mechanical system that obeys physical laws. Many of our postural and balance control mechanisms, essential for even the most basic activities, operate outside of conscious awareness. When these mechanisms break down—as in slipping or losing balance—we are rudely reminded of our physical limitations [1].

In the realm of physical ergonomics, understanding anatomy is crucial for designing work environments that promote health and efficiency. At its core, physical ergonomics focuses on how our bodies interact with the tools, equipment, and workspaces we use daily. To grasp how to optimize these interactions, one must first appreciate the intricate structure of the human body and how it responds to different physical demands. Our bodies are marvelously complex systems composed of bones, muscles, joints, and connective tissues, all working in harmony to support movement and stability. Bones provide the framework, muscles generate movement, and joints facilitate the range of motion. Connective tissues, such as tendons and ligaments, play a vital role in linking muscles to bones and stabilizing joints. When considering ergonomic design, the alignment and function of these anatomical components are paramount. For instance, the spine, which runs from the base of the skull to the pelvis, is a key player in maintaining posture. An ergonomic workstation should support the natural curvature of the spine, minimizing strain and preventing discomfort. This involves designing chairs and desks that allow for proper alignment, ensuring that the back is well supported and that the body is positioned to avoid undue stress. Muscles, too, are central to ergonomic considerations. Repetitive motions or sustained positions can lead to muscle fatigue and strain. Ergonomic solutions often involve redesigning tasks or tools to reduce the strain on specific muscle groups. For example, tools with ergonomic handles can decrease the strain on the hands and wrists, while adjustable workstations can help distribute physical effort more evenly. Joints are another critical focus in ergonomics. These are the points where bones meet and allow for movement. Poor ergonomics can place excessive stress on joints, leading to conditions such as carpal tunnel syndrome or tendinitis. By designing workspaces that allow for natural and comfortable movements, ergonomic interventions help prevent such injuries. The interplay between these anatomical elements and ergonomic design highlights the importance of a holistic approach to workplace design. When ergonomics is thoughtfully integrated, it considers not only the static aspects of body structure but also the dynamic aspects of movement and interaction. This comprehensive understanding helps in creating environments that support the body's natural functions, reduce the risk of injury, and enhance overall comfort and efficiency.

The word "anthropometry" is derived from the Greek words "Anthropos" (man) and "Metron" (measure), and means measurement of the human body. Anthropometric data are used in HFE to specify the physical dimensions of workspaces, equipment, vehicles, and clothing to ensure that these products physically fit the target population [1]. In the intricate dance of designing workspaces and tools, anthropometry plays a pivotal role, blending science with practicality to tailor environments to human needs. Anthropometry, the study of human body dimensions and their variations, serves as a foundation for creating ergonomic solutions that fit the diverse range of body sizes and shapes encountered in everyday life. Imagine stepping into a well-designed workspace where every element—from the height of the chair to the reach of the controls—is intuitively suited to your body. This seamless integration of design and body dimensions is the essence of anthropometry in ergonomics. By understanding the measurements and proportions of the human body, designers can craft environments that enhance comfort and efficiency while minimizing the risk of strain or injury. Anthropometry encompasses a range of measurements, including height, arm length, leg length, and various body circumferences. These dimensions are not uniform across the population; they vary widely among individuals. For example, consider the difference in stature between a tall person and a shorter one. An ergonomic chair that is adjustable in height and seat depth ensures that both can achieve a comfortable sitting posture, with their feet flat on the ground and their knees aligned with their hips. In practical terms, anthropometric data inform the design of everything from office furniture to industrial machinery. For instance, the height of a desk should be adjustable to accommodate different users, allowing for an optimal position where elbows rest comfortably at a 90-degree angle. Similarly, the reach of a control panel in a vehicle or machinery should be within easy access for operators of various sizes, reducing the need for awkward stretching or bending. The application of anthropometric principles is not merely about fitting the average user but also about accommodating a broad range of body types. This inclusive approach ensures that ergonomic solutions are accessible and comfortable for as many people as possible. By considering the extremes of body dimensions, designers can create adjustable and flexible systems that cater to individual needs.

2.1.2 Biomechanics

Biomechanics in ergonomics refers to the application of mechanical principles to the study of human movement and interaction with tools, equipment, and workspaces. It involves analyzing how forces and motions affect the human body, with the goal of designing environments and systems that align with the body's natural mechanical functions. By understanding the mechanical interactions between the body and its environment, biomechanics in ergonomics aims to optimize comfort, efficiency, and safety, reducing the risk of injury and improving overall performance. In the landscape of physical ergonomics, biomechanics is the key to understanding how our bodies move and respond to different forces. This branch of science delves into the mechanical aspects of human movement, exploring how forces and motions interact with our muscles, bones, and joints. Imagine biomechanics as the study of how our body acts like a complex machine. Each movement we make, whether it's lifting a heavy load or simply reaching for a file, involves a delicate balance of forces. These forces include gravity, muscle contractions, and the resistance provided by the objects we handle. Biomechanics examines how these elements come together, influencing our physical performance and comfort. One of the fundamental concepts in biomechanics is the idea of force distribution. For instance, when you lift an object, different muscles and joints are engaged to handle the weight. The biomechanics of lifting focuses on how to distribute this load efficiently to avoid overloading any single part of the body, thereby reducing the risk of injury. Improper lifting techniques can place excessive strain on the back and shoulders, leading to discomfort and long-term damage. In the context of ergonomics, applying biomechanical principles means designing tools and workspaces that align with how our bodies naturally move and function. For example, an ergonomic chair is not just about comfort; it's designed based on biomechanical principles to support proper posture and reduce strain on the back and neck. Similarly, the height and angle of a workstation are adjusted to ensure that tasks are performed in a way that minimizes mechanical stress on the body. Consider the example of a factory worker who spends hours using a hand tool. Biomechanics helps in designing this tool to fit comfortably in the hand, reducing the force required to operate it and minimizing the risk of repetitive strain injuries. The tool's design is informed by an understanding of how forces are transmitted through the hand and arm during use. By applying biomechanical insights, ergonomics creates work environments and tools that are not only efficient but also aligned with the body's mechanical capabilities. This approach helps prevent injuries, enhances performance, and improves overall comfort by ensuring that our physical interactions with the environment are well balanced and natural.

2.1.3 Physiology

Physiology in ergonomics is the study of how the body's physiological processes and systems respond to physical work and environmental conditions. It focuses on understanding how factors, such as muscle fatigue, cardiovascular response, and thermal regulation, affect human performance and comfort. In ergonomics, physiology helps to design work environments and tasks that align with the body's natural functions, optimizing efficiency, reducing strain, and preventing work-related health issues. At the heart of this understanding is how our muscles work during physical exertion. When you perform repetitive or strenuous tasks, muscles generate force and endurance. This continuous effort can lead to muscle fatigue and strain, if not managed properly. Ergonomic design uses this physiological insight to create tools and workspaces that minimize excessive muscle use and distribute physical effort more evenly. For example, ergonomic tools with contoured handles reduce the strain on the hands and wrists, while adjustable workstations allow for a range of postures that prevent overuse injuries. Cardiovascular responses are another critical focus. When engaging in physical work, the heart pumps more blood to meet the increased demand for oxygen and nutrients by the muscles. Prolonged or intense physical activity can place additional strain on the cardiovascular system. Ergonomic practices that include appropriate work-rest schedules and encourage movement can help mitigate this strain. By designing tasks and work environments that allow for periodic breaks and moderate activity levels, we can support cardiovascular health and enhance overall performance. Thermoregulation, the body's process of maintaining a stable internal temperature, is also influenced by ergonomic design. In varying temperature conditions, the body works to balance heat production and heat loss. In hot environments, sweat production increases to cool the body, while in cold conditions, the body generates heat through shivering and increased metabolic activity. Ergonomic solutions might involve providing adequate ventilation, cooling systems, or appropriate clothing to help the body regulate temperature effectively, ensuring comfort and preventing heat stress or hypothermia. Additionally, ergonomic design takes into account the body's natural rhythms and needs. For instance, the physiological need for rest and recovery is factored into work schedules to prevent fatigue and overuse injuries. Regular breaks, task rotation, and adjustments in workload help manage physical strain and support sustained productivity and well-being.

2.1.4 Workstation and workplace design

Workstation design involves arranging the physical elements of a workstation to promote good posture, reduce excessive movements, and ensure comfort. Key aspects include:

2.1.4.1 Adjustable furniture

Adjustable furniture in ergonomics refers to furniture designed to accommodate a wide range of human body sizes, postures, and preferences **Figure 1**. The idea behind adjustable furniture is to provide users with the ability to change the height, angle, or position of furniture to suit their personal needs, which improves comfort, reduces strain, and enhances productivity. In our daily lives, adjustable furniture plays a key role in promoting better health and well-being. For example, adjustable office chairs

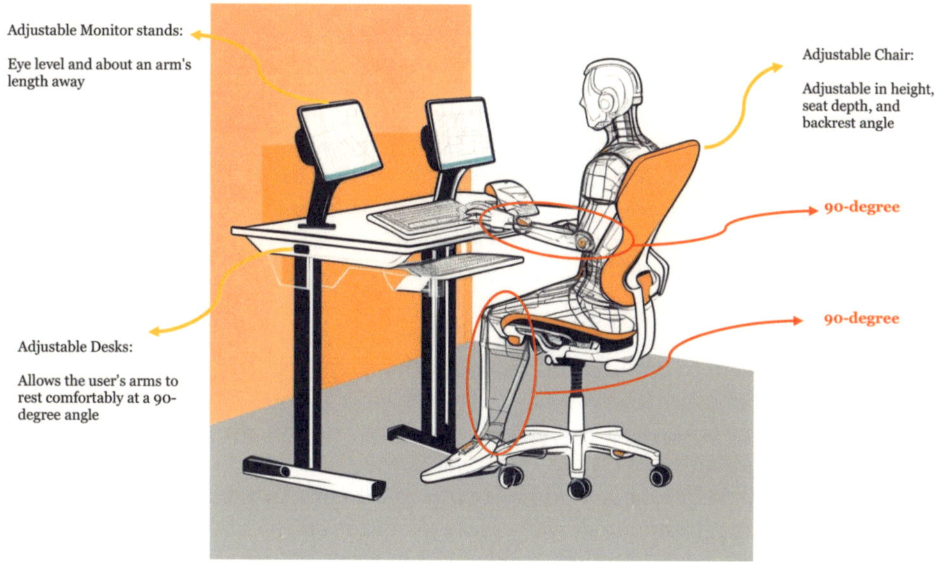

Figure 1.
Ergonomically designed adjustable furniture, including chairs, desks, and monitor stands, supports optimal posture and reduces the risk of musculoskeletal disorders by allowing users to customize their workspace.

and height-adjustable desks allow individuals to modify their workspace for optimal posture. This helps prevent back pain, neck strain, and carpal tunnel syndrome, which are common in people who spend long hours sitting at a desk. For example, in the home environment, adjustable furniture, such as reclining chairs or adjustable beds, provides comfort while performing various activities like watching TV, reading, or sleeping. These pieces help reduce physical stress and improve overall comfort. Furthermore, in educational settings, adjustable furniture has become increasingly important as schools realize the significance of ergonomic design. Adjustable desks and chairs can be tailored to the height and posture of students, ensuring they maintain good posture during long hours of study. This reduces discomfort and helps improve focus and learning outcomes. In growing children, furniture that adapts to their bodies reduces the risk of developing posture-related issues like scoliosis. Also, in hospitals and healthcare environments, ergonomically designed furniture is critical for both patients and healthcare workers. For patients, adjustable hospital beds and chairs enhance comfort and facilitate movement, making it easier for caregivers to provide care. For healthcare workers, adjustable workstations reduce the physical strain of bending or lifting, leading to fewer injuries and a more efficient workflow. In modern workplaces, adjustable furniture is crucial for maintaining the health and productivity of office workers. Spending long hours sitting at a desk can lead to various physical issues, such as back pain, neck strain, and wrist discomfort, especially when the furniture does not fit the user's body properly. Ergonomically designed adjustable furniture offers solutions to these problems by allowing individuals to modify their workspace to fit their unique needs.

Chairs: Ergonomic chairs should be adjustable in height, seat depth, and backrest angle. This allows users to maintain a neutral posture where the feet are flat on the floor, knees are at a 90-degree angle, and the back is supported. Features, such as lumbar support, padded armrests, and a seat with a slightly forward tilt, can reduce lower back strain and improve comfort.

Desks: Desks should be at an appropriate height that allows the user's arms to rest comfortably at a 90-degree angle. Adjustable desks, particularly sit-stand desks, provide the flexibility to alternate between sitting and standing positions, reducing the risk of musculoskeletal disorders associated with prolonged sitting or standing.

Monitor stands: Monitors should be positioned at eye level and about an arm's length away to reduce neck strain. Adjustable monitor stands allow users to customize the height and angle of the screen, helping to maintain a neutral neck posture and reduce eye strain.

2.1.5 Layout and organization

In ergonomics, refer to the integrated approach of designing and arranging the physical environment to optimize human performance, comfort, and safety. Together, these principles aim to create a workspace that supports the user's physical and cognitive needs, reducing strain and enhancing efficiency. Some of the most important components are explained below:

Reach zones: Workstations should be organized into primary, secondary, and tertiary reach zones to minimize awkward postures and excessive reaching. Frequently used items (primary reach zone) should be within arm's length, while less frequently used items (secondary and tertiary reach zones) should be placed further away. This reduces the need for excessive bending, twisting, and reaching, lowering the risk of repetitive strain injuries.

Clearance and space: Adequate space should be provided for leg movement and freedom of movement around the workstation. This includes proper clearance for knees and feet under the desk and enough space around the workstation for easy access and movement.

Organizing the workspace: A crucial aspect of designing a productive and comfortable work environment. It involves arranging the physical environment to align with ergonomic principles, ensuring that tools, materials, and furniture are positioned to support user comfort, efficiency, and safety. Effective organization reduces physical strain, enhances productivity, and promotes a healthier and more enjoyable work experience.

2.1.6 Environmental ergonomics

Environmental ergonomics focuses on optimizing the physical environment to improve human health, comfort, and performance, especially in workplaces. This field examines the interaction between individuals and environmental factors, such as lighting, temperature, noise, humidity, and air quality. Environmental ergonomics aims to design settings that prevent discomfort, reduce stress, and minimize health risks, which can lead to better productivity and well-being.

Environmental ergonomics indeed considers both external environmental factors (like lighting, temperature, humidity, noise, and air quality) and internal environmental factors (such as psychological and physiological conditions that affect comfort, health, and performance).

2.1.6.1 Lighting

The overall lighting in the workplace should be adequate for the tasks being performed. Ambient lighting should provide sufficient illumination without causing glare or shadows, while task-specific lighting should address the needs of detailed or precision work.

Intensity: Lighting should be bright enough to avoid eye strain but not so intense as to cause glare.

Color temperature: The color temperature (measured in Kelvin) affects visual comfort. For instance, cool white light (4000–5000 K) is often preferred for workspaces, while warmer light (2700–3000 K) is used in relaxation areas.

Glare control: Minimize glare from direct light sources and reflective surfaces by using diffusers or shades.

2.1.6.2 Temperature and humidity

Maintaining a comfortable temperature and humidity level is essential for worker comfort and efficiency. Extremes in temperature can lead to discomfort, fatigue, and reduced concentration. Proper ventilation and climate control systems help maintain a stable and comfortable environment.

2.1.6.2.1 Temperature regulation

Comfort: Maintaining a comfortable temperature range (generally between 20 and 22°C or between 68 and 72°F) is essential for productivity and comfort. Extreme temperatures can cause discomfort and reduce performance.

Health: Prolonged exposure to extreme cold or heat can lead to health issues, such as hypothermia, heat exhaustion, or heat stroke.

2.1.6.2.2 Temperature control measures

Ventilation: Ensure adequate airflow to maintain a consistent temperature and remove stale air.

Heating and cooling systems: Use air conditioning, heaters, or fans to regulate temperature based on the needs of the workspace.

Personal comfort: Provide options for individuals to adjust their immediate environment, such as adjustable fans or personal heaters.

2.1.6.2.3 Impact of humidity

Comfort and health: High humidity can make temperatures feel warmer and cause discomfort, while low humidity can lead to dry skin, respiratory issues, and static electricity.

Equipment performance: Excessive humidity can affect electronic equipment and materials, leading to malfunction or damage.

2.1.6.2.4 Humidity control

Dehumidifiers and humidifiers: Use devices to maintain optimal humidity levels (generally between 30 and 50%).

Ventilation: Ensure proper ventilation to manage humidity levels and prevent condensation and mold growth.

2.1.6.3 Noise control

Excessive noise can lead to stress, reduced concentration, and communication difficulties. Acoustic treatments, such as sound-absorbing materials and partitions, can reduce noise levels and create a more conducive working environment.

Sound absorption: Use materials that absorb sound, such as acoustic panels, carpets, and curtains, to reduce noise levels.

Sound barriers: Install partitions or barriers to block or deflect noise from high-traffic or noisy areas.

White noise: Introduce background white noise to mask disruptive sounds and create a more consistent acoustic environment.

2.1.6.4 Ergonomic signage and safety for risk reduction

- *Signage:* Clear, ergonomic signage is critical for reducing workplace accidents and enhancing overall safety. Signs should be positioned at eye level to avoid strain and increase visibility, use large, easily readable fonts, and incorporate universal symbols, wherever possible. These factors help ensure workers quickly comprehend important instructions, minimizing risks associated with confusion or misinterpretation.

- *Emergency exits and safety equipment:* Clearly marked and accessible emergency exits and safety equipment are essential to preventing injuries in emergencies. Exit routes should be unobstructed, and safety equipment, such as fire extinguishers and first aid kits, should be easily accessible and routinely inspected to ensure functionality. This proactive approach reduces risk by providing prompt access to resources in critical moments.

2.1.6.5 Break areas and rest zones for risk mitigation

- *Dedicated break areas:* Establishing comfortable, quiet break areas supports physical and mental recovery, reducing fatigue-related errors and injuries. Equipped with amenities like comfortable seating, water dispensers, coffee machines, and snack options, these areas offer workers a proper setting for rest, ultimately enhancing alertness and performance.

- *Rest zones for recovery:* In physically demanding roles, rest zones equipped with reclining chairs, stretch areas, or even massage stations enable workers to recover effectively from physical strain. By promoting muscle relaxation and addressing fatigue, these spaces are instrumental in lowering the risk of musculoskeletal disorders and other strain-related injuries.

2.2 Cognitive ergonomics

Cognitive ergonomics is a branch of the broader field of ergonomics, also known as human factors. It focuses on designing systems, tasks, and environments in a way that aligns with human mental abilities and limitations. Essentially, it's about making sure that the interaction between people and their work, the products they use, and the environments they are in are well suited to human needs and capabilities, while also considering their limitations. In this interaction between humans and systems, cognitive ergonomics zeroes in on how our minds work. It specifically looks at mental processes, such as thinking, reasoning, and decision-making, as well as the psychological and behavioral ways we interact with systems and environments. This area is all about fine-tuning these interactions to boost human performance while lightening the mental load. By doing so, it helps cut down on mistakes and enhances safety.

Cognitive ergonomics, often called cognitive engineering, uses scientific insights into human behavior, abilities, and limitations to make cognitive tasks more efficient [2]. It highlights the importance of cognitive processes like perception, attention, learning, memory, and decision-making. These mental functions play a crucial role, especially in complex and constantly shifting environments where the cognitive workload is high [3]. In the brain, cognitive processes take place simultaneously, driven by the interactions of around 100 billion neurons and countless neurotransmitters working together [3]. While physical ergonomics deals with more visible factors like posture and muscle strain, cognitive ergonomics focuses on the less obvious aspects of how we process information and complete tasks. In high-pressure situations, for instance, perception often leads straight to action without much thought. But at other times, we actively engage with the information we perceive, combining it with what we already know through working memory (WM). WM is where we hold the information we are actively thinking about—whether it's something we have just perceived or retrieved from long-term memory (LTM). It's the space for conscious activities like planning, decision-making, understanding, visualizing, rehearsing, and problem-solving. However, WM has limited capacity, holding information only for a short time, unless we transfer it into LTM [3, 4]. Since working memory (WM) is temporary, keeping information active within it demands focused attention. As we concentrate on it, manipulate it, and rehearse it, some of the information in WM becomes encoded into long-term memory (LTM), where it can be accessed later. This process is what we call learning [3]. To truly understand cognitive ergonomics, one must recognize the delicate balance it maintains. Humans are remarkable in their ability to handle complex information, but there are limits. The mind, like any system, can be overloaded, distracted, or fatigued. Cognitive ergonomics aims to reduce this load by designing work environments, tools, and processes that work with, rather than against, human cognitive abilities. Whether it's ensuring that controls are intuitive, alarms are distinguishable, or information is presented in a digestible format, the goal remains the same: to minimize errors and maximize efficiency by respecting the capabilities and limitations of the human mind. This focus on mental processing extends beyond the individual and into the interaction between people. Collaboration in teams, for instance, can be influenced by how information is shared, understood, and acted upon. Cognitive ergonomics considers how communication flows, how decision-making is distributed, and how shared knowledge can be leveraged to improve group performance. In high-stakes environments like air traffic control, surgery, or emergency response, the importance of getting these elements right cannot be overstated.

2.2.1 Key focus areas in cognitive ergonomics

2.2.1.1 Sensation and perception

Sensation and perception form the foundation upon which cognitive ergonomics builds its understanding of how humans interact with their environments. These two processes are often seen as inseparable, yet they play distinct roles in how we experience the world and, consequently, how we perform tasks within it. Sensation refers to the initial detection of stimuli through our sensory organs—the eyes, ears, skin, and so on. It is the raw data that our bodies collect from the external world, whether it's the brightness of a monitor, the sound of an alarm, or the texture of a tool. This is where the human body serves as a receptor, passively gathering information without yet assigning it meaning or context. In an ergonomic context, the design of workspaces and equipment must account for how sensory input is received. For example, if an alarm is too faint or a display too dim, the individual may not detect them adequately, potentially leading to serious consequences. Perception, on the other hand, is the process by which the brain interprets these sensory signals. It's not enough to simply see or hear; the brain must make sense of the input, drawing on past experiences, context, and cognitive processes to understand what is happening and how to respond. In many ways, perception transforms sensation into something meaningful. For instance, the worker hears a sound, but its perception that tells them it's an urgent alarm, not just background noise. Perception involves two key processes: bottom-up, where we analyze the physical characteristics of stimuli, and top-down, where our prior knowledge and expectations, drawn from long-term memory (LTM), come into play [3]. In cognitive ergonomics, the distinction between sensation and perception becomes critically important. Designers must account not only for whether a signal can be sensed but also for how it will be perceived under different conditions. This is particularly relevant in high-stress or high-stakes environments, where misperceptions can lead to errors. For example, in a cockpit, where numerous alarms, signals, and gauges are constantly vying for attention, cognitive ergonomics seeks to ensure that the most important information is not just detected but immediately understood. If a pilot misperceives an alarm due to its tone or timing, the result could be catastrophic. Sensation and perception are also affected by the context in which they occur. Fatigue, stress, and distractions can alter how we sense and perceive the world around us. A fatigued worker might fail to notice subtle cues in their environment, while someone under pressure might misinterpret those same cues due to the cognitive load they are experiencing. This is where cognitive ergonomics steps in to mitigate such risks by designing environments that are less taxing on our sensory and perceptual systems. For instance, color-coded displays, distinct sound alerts, and carefully structured workflows can help ensure that critical information is both sensed and perceived correctly, even under challenging conditions. An understanding that human beings are not perfect machines; our senses can fail us, and our perceptions can be distorted. But by recognizing these limitations, we can create systems that enhance our natural abilities, reducing the likelihood of errors and improving overall performance. Sensation and perception involve how we interpret stimuli received through our senses—like sight, hearing, taste, smell, or touch. For example, in construction, it's essential to hear warning signals, while in medical settings, recognizing symbols on a monitor is critical.

2.2.1.2 Attention

Attention is the stage where we concentrate on specific elements of the information we perceive, or sometimes divide our focus among multiple aspects. For instance, in a control room, it's crucial to recognize if there has been a significant change in the situation. Attention, in the context of cognitive ergonomics, is a critical aspect of how humans interact with their environment, tasks, and tools. It is the mental process that enables us to focus selectively on certain stimuli while ignoring others, guiding us through the immense amount of information we encounter at any given moment. Understanding attention is key to designing systems, workplaces, and tools that align with the way our mind's function, ensuring that we can perform tasks efficiently and safely. Attention is not a singular, fixed process; it is fluid and can be divided, shifted, or sustained depending on the demands of the situation. When a person concentrates on a particular task, such as operating complex machinery or monitoring multiple screens in a control room, their ability to maintain focus is vital to the accuracy and speed of their actions. However, attention is a finite resource. It can be overwhelmed by too many stimuli, fatigued by prolonged periods of concentration, or fragmented when trying to multitask. This is where cognitive ergonomics plays a crucial role—designing environments and systems that do not overload our attentional capacity but rather support and enhance it. One of the primary challenges in attention is the balance between focused attention and divided attention. Focused attention allows us to zero in on a specific task or piece of information, filtering out distractions. This might occur when a surgeon performs a delicate procedure or when a worker is analyzing a complex dataset. In these scenarios, distractions must be minimized to ensure that attention is not diverted from the critical task at hand. Cognitive ergonomics seeks to reduce unnecessary noise—whether literal, visual, or informational—so that focused attention can be sustained effectively. Divided attention, on the other hand, is the ability to manage multiple tasks or sources of information simultaneously. While humans are not inherently great multitaskers, certain jobs require us to balance multiple inputs. For example, a pilot must simultaneously monitor the controls, communicate with air traffic control, and make adjustments based on changing weather conditions. Cognitive ergonomics helps design these multitasking environments to ensure that the division of attention does not lead to information overload or errors. Thoughtful placement of controls, clear visual hierarchy, and prioritized alerts all serve to guide attention in a manageable way. Moreover, attention is dynamic and can be influenced by various factors, such as fatigue, stress, or repetitive tasks. When people are fatigued, their ability to maintain attention diminishes, increasing the likelihood of mistakes or accidents. In high-pressure environments, attention may become overly fixated on certain details while missing others—a phenomenon known as "tunnel vision." Cognitive ergonomics aims to combat these risks by designing systems that either alleviate the mental burden or prompt shifts in attention as needed. For example, timed breaks or automated alerts can be incorporated into workflows to remind workers to refocus or rest.

Ultimately, attention in cognitive ergonomics is about guiding the user's mental resources efficiently and effectively. It's about recognizing the limitations of human attention and designing systems that complement rather than challenge those limits. Whether the task requires deep concentration or multitasking, understanding how attention works allows us to create environments that keep people engaged, alert, and—above all—safe.

2.2.1.3 Working memory

Working memory encompasses a short-term storage system where information can be held for up to 30 seconds. It also involves the mental processes used to actively rehearse and manipulate that information. Working memory (WM) temporarily holds active information, whether it's perceived from our surroundings or retrieved from long-term memory (LTM). It keeps this information accessible for a short period while we use it or until we transfer it into LTM [5]. While in working memory (WM), information can be utilized and manipulated by various cognitive processes like planning, reasoning, and decision-making. However, WM can typically hold only about four chunks of information for a limited duration [6]. A chunk serves as a unit of working memory (WM) space, consisting of information grouped together by meaning—like relatedness, similarity, familiarity, or cooccurrence. By combining multiple items into a single chunk, it reduces the total number of individual pieces in WM, effectively increasing its capacity [3]. Working memory, in the field of cognitive ergonomics, is a crucial mental function that allows us to temporarily hold and manipulate information while performing tasks. It is like the brain's mental workspace, where relevant information is actively processed to solve problems, make decisions, or complete complex activities. Working memory is not a storage system but a dynamic, short-term tool that helps us carry out immediate tasks by keeping necessary information at the forefront of our minds. In the context of cognitive ergonomics, understanding the limits of working memory is essential for designing systems and tasks that align with human capabilities. Our working memory is limited in both capacity and duration. Typically, we can hold only a small amount of information—about seven items, give or take, depending on the individual—for a short period of time. This means that when we are overloaded with too much information at once, or asked to juggle multiple pieces of data simultaneously, the chances of errors, omissions, or confusion increase. Cognitive ergonomics seeks to design environments that reduce this cognitive load, ensuring that tasks can be performed accurately without overburdening the worker's mental resources. Consider a scenario in a control room, where an operator must keep track of numerous indicators, alarms, and ongoing processes. If too much information is presented simultaneously, the operator's working memory could quickly become overwhelmed. This is where ergonomic principles come into play. By organizing information in a logical and manageable manner—perhaps through chunking related pieces of data together, using visual aids, or prioritizing critical alerts—the operator's working memory can function more effectively. The goal is to ensure that the mental effort required to hold and use this information does not exceed the natural capacity of the mind. Working memory is also involved in multitasking and decision-making. In environments where tasks require rapid shifts in focus or the integration of multiple streams of information, it is vital that systems are designed to support these processes. For example, in air traffic control, a controller must monitor aircraft positions, communicate with pilots, and manage unforeseen events—all of which rely on an efficient working memory. When designed properly, interfaces and tools can offload some of this cognitive burden by externalizing information or prompting the controller at the right moments, helping to conserve mental resources. Fatigue, stress, and distractions can further impair working memory. As cognitive load increases, the brain struggles to maintain focus and retain important information, leading to a higher risk of mistakes. Cognitive ergonomics aims to mitigate this by designing environments that support working memory through simplicity, clarity, and well-timed interventions. For instance, systems can be designed to offer reminders or visual prompts, ensuring that essential information is not lost in the shuffle of competing tasks.

In sum, working memory plays a vital role in how we process and use information in real time. Cognitive ergonomics acknowledges its limitations and strives to create environments where tasks are not overwhelming, where information is presented in digestible amounts, and where the mental workload (MWL) is kept within manageable bounds. This focus ensures that workers can operate efficiently and make decisions with clarity, even in fast-paced or high-stress situations.

2.2.1.4 Long-term memory

Long-term memory (LTM) acts as a permanent storage system for various types of information. Semantic memory involves knowledge about the world, including symbols and concepts. Episodic memory holds information about specific events and experiences, while autobiographical memories pertain to significant moments in an individual's personal life. Additionally, procedural knowledge relates to "knowing how" to perform tasks and skills. LTM serves as the mechanism for learning new information, temporarily storing it, and allowing for later retrieval [7]. There are three types of long-term memory (LTM): (1) Semantic memory, which contains factual knowledge—like the difference between afferent and efferent nerves; (2) Episodic memory, which involves knowledge of specific events—such as your first day at work; and (3) Procedural memory, which encompasses the knowledge of how to perform tasks—like properly intubating a patient. LTM is organized based on meaning, with related items being stored closer together than unrelated ones [3]. One theory of long-term memory (LTM) suggests that knowledge is organized through semantic networks, where concepts are represented as nodes and the relationships between these concepts are depicted as links [8]. In these networks, closely related concepts are directly linked, while unrelated concepts are distanced by multiple links. Another perspective on knowledge organization is through schemas [9]. Schemas represent a theme or central topic connected to the information stored in long-term memory (LTM). When schemas outline a typical sequence of activities, they are referred to as scripts. For example, you might have a script for taking a patient's medical history [3]. Prospective memory refers to the ability to remember to carry out a task or intention in the future [10]. Environmental reminders and checklists can help enhance prospective memory [11]. Additionally, verbally stating intentions or taking physical actions can enhance prospective memory. It's also crucial to recognize how people forget. Typically, individuals forget what they have learned quickly, following an exponential curve, with significant forgetting occurring within the first few days [12]. For this reason, assessing the effects of training immediately after instruction does not accurately reflect the extent of an individual's eventual memory retention. Additionally, various forms of long-term memory (LTM) retrieval decline at different rates. Specifically, recall, which requires actively retrieving the needed information, tends to fade more quickly than recognition, where a perceptual cue is present in the environment [3]. Long-term memory, in the context of cognitive ergonomics, serves as the mental archive where information is stored over extended periods, ranging from days to decades. It is through long-term memory that individuals retain knowledge, skills, experiences, and patterns, which they can retrieve when needed for decision-making, problem-solving, or performing tasks. Unlike working memory, which handles information temporarily and is limited in capacity, long-term memory is vast, capable of holding an incredible amount of data for indefinite periods. In cognitive ergonomics, long-term memory is significant because it provides the foundation for expertise, familiarity with tasks, and the recognition of patterns. When workers are performing tasks that rely on procedures learned over time, they draw heavily on their long-term memory. This could be the case for a surgeon recalling the steps of a procedure, a pilot remembering how to respond to specific flight conditions, or an engineer troubleshooting a recurring system error. The efficiency with which individuals retrieve and apply this stored information can influence their performance, especially in high-stakes or complex environments. Designing for long-term memory in cognitive ergonomics involves supporting how information is encoded, stored, and retrieved. Tasks and systems should be designed to facilitate easy learning and retention, ensuring that important information can move into long-term memory more effectively. One of the key ways to achieve this is through repetition and practice, which reinforce the neural pathways associated with a specific skill or body of knowledge. Over time, this process allows workers to perform tasks more automatically, reducing the cognitive effort required and freeing up working memory for more immediate or complex decision-making. Retrieval from long-term memory can be influenced by cues in the environment. For example, visual or auditory signals, specific words, or even the layout of a workspace can trigger the recall of important information or procedures. Cognitive ergonomics seeks to design these cues in a way that supports fast and accurate retrieval. Consider a control room where different colored alarms correspond to specific types of system failures; these visual cues help operators quickly recall the appropriate response based on past training. Similarly, the use of consistent, familiar symbols or terms in a user interface can prompt the recall of how a task is performed, allowing workers to act efficiently without having to consciously think through each step. However, long-term memory is not infallible. It is subject to forgetting, distortion, or interference from new information. Cognitive ergonomics addresses these limitations by designing systems that compensate for memory lapses. For instance, checklists, procedural guides, or automated reminders can be integrated into workflows, ensuring that critical steps are not overlooked, even if an individual's memory fails them in the moment. By recognizing that long-term memory, while powerful, is not perfect, cognitive ergonomics provides safeguards to minimize the impact of memory errors.

So, long-term memory plays an important role in how people perform tasks that rely on accumulated knowledge and expertise. In cognitive ergonomics, understanding the role of long-term memory allows designers to create environments that reinforce learning, support accurate recall, and reduce the likelihood of mistakes due to memory failures. This approach not only enhances performance but also contributes to safety and efficiency in complex work environments.

2.2.1.5 Learning

Learning, at its core, is the process through which individuals acquire new knowledge, skills, or behaviors, and adapt them to their experiences and environments. It is a continuous and dynamic journey, deeply rooted in the human capacity to observe, understand, and internalize information, ultimately transforming how one interacts with the world. Whether it is conscious or subconscious, intentional or incidental, learning influences every aspect of cognition, shaping not only what people know, but how they think and solve problems. In the context of cognitive ergonomics, learning becomes more than just a passive intake of information; it is an active process where individuals refine their mental processes and build cognitive structures that allow them to navigate tasks and environments with increasing ease and efficiency. Here, learning is intertwined with the adaptation of the brain to complex systems and workflows, often driven by the need to reduce cognitive load and minimize the risk of errors in high-stakes situations. Learning, in this sense, is cumulative. It builds on past experiences, allowing the mind to create mental shortcuts, anticipate outcomes, and make decisions more fluidly over time. This progression is central to the design of ergonomic systems that support human cognition, as they must account for how individuals learn and how that learning impacts their ability to perform tasks safely and effectively. People often simplify the complexity of the material they learn by organizing items into categories, particularly hierarchical ones [13]. For instance, user interfaces that group related items together tend to be easier to learn compared to those that do not [14]. This arrangement offers hints about the underlying model of the device. Moreover, individuals naturally look for similarities between new situations and past experiences. As a result, learning is often enhanced through the use of analogy and metaphor [15]. Devices are generally easier to learn when they maintain consistency in labeling, information placement, and color coding [16].

2.2.1.6 Decision-making

Decision-making involves choosing an option from various alternatives, particularly when risk and uncertainty are present. For about the last 40 years, research primarily concentrated on how people ought to make decisions rather than how they actually do. Recently, however, psychologists and economists have started to explore how real individuals make real choices. These two perspectives are known as normative and descriptive decision-making, and they lead to very different insights. Making decisions requires evaluating multiple options, each associated with different probabilities of outcomes, as well as their respective strengths and weaknesses. While computers excel at managing these factors and performing calculations simultaneously, people struggle with this task. Unlike computers, individuals have limited perception, working memory (WM), and attentional resources. As a result, they often rely on shortcuts known as heuristics "rules of thumb" that enable them to make satisfactory rather than optimal decisions [3]. Choosing shortcuts and settling on a decision that is "good enough," instead of evaluating all possible options, is referred to as satisficing [17]. When satisficing, the decision-maker creates and assesses options only until they find one that is acceptable, rather than seeking the optimal choice. This approach is effective, given that individuals have limited cognitive capacities and time [18]. Decision-making in the context of cognitive ergonomics is a critical function that reflects the way individuals process information, assess situations, and ultimately select a course of action. It is a cognitive activity where the mind navigates through options, weighing risks and benefits, while being influenced by numerous internal and external factors. The complexity of decision-making is rooted in the mental processes that allow individuals to filter through vast amounts of information, prioritize relevant data, and formulate a choice that aligns with the objectives or constraints of the environment they are operating in. In cognitive ergonomics, decision-making is not merely about choosing between options; it is about optimizing the conditions under which decisions are made. This involves understanding how people perceive their environments, how they process information under varying levels of stress or complexity, and how their cognitive limits affect their ability to make sound judgments. Decision-making, in this sense, is influenced by both the quality of the information available and the mental capacity of the individual to process that information efficiently. It is here that cognitive ergonomics plays a vital role, designing systems that reduce unnecessary cognitive load and ensure that the information needed for decision-making is both accessible and comprehensible. A fundamental aspect of decision-making is the reliance on mental models—internal representations that individuals create based on experience and knowledge. These models help individuals predict the outcomes of their decisions and guide them through uncertain or complex situations. Cognitive ergonomics seeks to support this process by designing environments and systems that align with these mental models, reducing the effort required to make decisions and, in turn, improving overall performance. Furthermore, decision-making in cognitive ergonomics is closely tied to how individuals respond to feedback. Feedback loops play a significant role in refining future decisions, as they allow individuals to learn from past choices and adjust their strategies accordingly. In well-designed ergonomic systems, feedback is provided in real time, ensuring that the decision-making process is continuously informed by the outcomes of previous actions. This dynamic adjustment helps to mitigate risks and reduce errors, as individuals are better equipped to recognize when they need to reconsider their approach or adapt to new circumstances. In high-risk environments, where decision-making can have immediate and severe consequences, cognitive ergonomics emphasizes the importance of minimizing distractions and streamlining the flow of information to aid in faster, more accurate decision-making. Here, the balance between speed and accuracy becomes crucial. Cognitive ergonomics addresses this by designing tools and interfaces that allow individuals to make decisions with confidence, even under pressure, by ensuring that their cognitive resources are used efficiently.

To summarize, decision-making in cognitive ergonomics is about facilitating human interaction with systems and environments in a way that enhances judgment, reduces the likelihood of error, and supports the continuous learning process. It is a deeply cognitive function that reflects how well individuals are equipped to navigate the complexities of their tasks, and how effectively the systems they interact with support their ability to make informed, timely, and appropriate decisions.

2.2.1.7 Mental workload

Mental workload in cognitive ergonomics pertains to the cognitive demands imposed on an individual during task performance. It includes the amount of mental effort needed to complete a task, how that effort impacts performance, and the overall implications for well-being and efficiency. Recognizing and managing mental workload is essential for designing systems, interfaces, and tasks that enhance performance while minimizing cognitive strain. Human mental workload is arguably one of the most referenced multidimensional constructs in Human Factors and Ergonomics, gaining traction in fields like Neuroscience and Neuroergonomics as well [19]. One of the main objectives of developing interactive technologies from a human factor's standpoint has consistently been to manage the mental workload (MWL) experienced by users. The key motivations behind this are to optimize their performance, enhance their engagement, and reduce errors. Every human activity involves some degree of mental processing, which means that there is always a certain level of mental workload involved [20]. Even the simplest physical or cognitive tasks require some level of mental processing, which in turn generates a certain degree of mental workload [21, 22]. The term "mental workload" is often used broadly to encompass the demands placed on users, the effort required by operators to meet those demands, and the outcomes of attempting to fulfill them [23]. Mental workload, within the framework of cognitive ergonomics, refers to the cognitive effort required for an individual to complete a task, process information, or make decisions within a given environment. It is a measure of the strain placed on a person's mental capacities when performing activities that demand attention, memory, reasoning, or problem-solving. Unlike physical workload, which pertains to the body's exertion, mental workload is focused on how the brain handles the complexities and pressures associated with a task, and how it manages the cognitive resources necessary to achieve a desired outcome. In cognitive ergonomics, the concept of mental workload is central to understanding human performance in work environments, especially those that require sustained concentration or the management of multiple streams of information. When the mental workload is balanced, individuals can perform their tasks with accuracy and efficiency, experiencing minimal cognitive strain. However, when the mental workload exceeds a person's capacity, it can lead to errors, fatigue, and a significant reduction in performance. This overload often occurs when tasks are too complex, too fast-paced, or require constant attention to a wide range of variables simultaneously, pushing cognitive limits to the breaking point. Cognitive ergonomics seeks to manage and optimize mental workload by designing systems, tools, and environments that align with the natural limits of human cognition. By reducing unnecessary cognitive demands, such as overly complex interfaces or excessive multitasking, the mental workload can be adjusted to a level where individuals can operate effectively without experiencing burnout or confusion. The goal is to ensure that the mental workload remains within a person's capacity to process information, make decisions, and take appropriate actions, all while maintaining a high level of performance and safety. An important element of mental workload in cognitive ergonomics is the recognition that individuals have different thresholds for handling mental strain. Factors, such as experience, familiarity with the task, the presence of external stressors, and even individual differences in cognitive abilities, all contribute to how mental workload is perceived and managed. As such, cognitive ergonomists must consider these variations when designing systems that accommodate a wide range of users, ensuring that mental workloads are distributed in a way that enhances performance rather than impeding it. Moreover, mental workload is not static; it fluctuates based on the demands of the task and the individual's ability to adapt to those demands. In environments where tasks become progressively more challenging or time-sensitive, mental workload can increase rapidly, leading to cognitive fatigue. This is why cognitive ergonomics emphasizes the importance of feedback and support systems that allow individuals to manage their workload more effectively. For example, clear and intuitive interfaces, timely feedback, and supportive tools can all help reduce the cognitive strain by guiding the user through their tasks and providing cues that aid in decision-making and information processing. In summary, mental workload in cognitive ergonomics is about balancing the cognitive demands placed on individuals with their mental capacity to handle those demands effectively. By understanding the intricacies of mental workload, cognitive ergonomists can design environments and systems that enhance human performance, reduce errors, and ensure that tasks are completed efficiently without overwhelming the brain's natural cognitive limits. This focus on mental workload is essential to creating safe, productive, and user-friendly workspaces where individuals can thrive without being mentally overburdened.

2.2.2 Implications of mental workload

2.2.2.1 Performance

Efficiency: High mental workload can lead to slower performance and increased error rates. Properly managing workload can enhance efficiency and accuracy.

Learning and adaptation: A manageable mental workload supports learning and adaptation, allowing users to develop skills and improve performance over time.

2.2.2.2 Well-being

Stress and health: Excessive mental workload can lead to stress, burnout, and mental fatigue. Managing workload effectively helps in maintaining mental health and well-being.

Job satisfaction: A well-designed task and interface that minimizes unnecessary cognitive demands can improve job satisfaction and overall work experience.

2.2.3 Applications in design

2.2.3.1 System design

Adaptive systems: Design systems that adapt to the user's level of expertise or current workload, providing more or less assistance as needed.

User-centered design: It focuses on the needs and capabilities of the user to design systems and tasks that align with their cognitive abilities.

2.2.4 Cognitive ergonomics research

Ongoing research: Current research on cognitive ergonomics focuses on enhancing human performance, safety, and efficiency across various high-stakes environments. Studies are exploring cognitive load management and human-automation interactions in fields like healthcare, aviation, and military settings, aiming to prevent overload and errors. Virtual and augmented reality (VR/AR) are being used to simulate hazardous tasks and assist in real time, while Artificial Intelligence (AI)-driven adaptive interfaces are designed to personalize information and reduce information overload in sectors like finance and emergency response. Another area of focus is the human-robot interaction, specifically with collaborative robots (cobots), where intuitive interfaces support shared control, ensuring safe and efficient task execution.

Research is also examining the cognitive impacts of remote work, aiming to reduce digital fatigue and improve productivity in mobile environments. Ongoing studies on healthcare interfaces focus on error detection, while autonomous vehicle research looks at enhancing driver readiness and trust in automated systems. Brain-computer interfaces (BCIs) for real-time cognitive monitoring are another innovative focus, especially valuable in roles requiring sustained attention, such as air traffic control and long-haul driving. Altogether, these efforts aim to leverage advanced technologies to create environments that support cognitive well-being, decision-making accuracy, and safety.

2.2.5 Human-computer interaction (HCI)

Human-computer interaction, or HCI, is a multidisciplinary field that explores how people engage with computers, digital systems, and technology, focusing on the design and usability of these interactions. In cognitive ergonomics, HCI plays a critical role, as it delves into how users mentally process and respond to the interfaces and systems they interact with. This interaction is not merely about inputting commands or navigating through software; it is fundamentally about the cognitive processes involved in understanding and using the technology to achieve specific goals. At its core, HCI within cognitive ergonomics seeks to create a seamless experience where the user can perform tasks with minimal cognitive strain. This requires designing interfaces that align with the way humans naturally perceive, think, and make decisions. The cognitive aspect of HCI considers how information is presented to the user, how easily it can be understood, and how the design can support memory, attention, and problem-solving skills. It is about making sure that the system complements the user's mental capabilities, rather than overwhelming them. In cognitive ergonomics, human-computer interaction is studied to enhance the ease with which users can learn, operate, and navigate a system. A key principle is the reduction of cognitive load, meaning that the design of a computer system should not burden the user with unnecessary complexities or overwhelming information. When interfaces are cluttered, unintuitive, or require excessive multitasking, they impose a higher cognitive load on the user, increasing the likelihood of errors, frustration, and fatigue. The goal, then, is to design systems that are clear, intuitive, and allow users to focus on the task at hand rather than on how to operate the system itself. One important concept in this interaction is usability, which refers to how easy and efficient it is for users to accomplish their tasks within a given system. From the perspective of cognitive ergonomics, usability is not just about functionality but about aligning the design with the mental models of users. Mental models are the internal representations people form based on their experiences, allowing them to predict how a system should behave. If a system aligns well with these models, the user can navigate it more naturally, with less cognitive effort. Another critical element of HCI within cognitive ergonomics is feedback. When users interact with a computer system, they rely on feedback to understand the outcomes of their actions and to adjust their behavior accordingly. This feedback must be timely, clear, and relevant to the user's actions. For example, visual or auditory cues that confirm an action has been completed successfully reduce uncertainty and help the user feel more in control. Cognitive ergonomics focuses on ensuring that such feedback enhances the user's understanding without overwhelming them or creating confusion. Human-computer interaction in cognitive ergonomics also examines how technology can support decision-making processes. As users often rely on computers to analyze information or assist in complex tasks, the system must present data in a way that supports critical thinking and problem-solving. This means not only offering the right information at the right time but doing so in a manner that is easy to interpret and act upon. Systems that can anticipate the user's needs or adapt to their behaviors help to streamline decision-making, further reducing cognitive load and enhancing performance. In environments where users must interact with complex or high-risk systems, such as in aviation or healthcare, the principles of HCI within cognitive ergonomics become even more critical. Here, the stakes are high, and any inefficiency or confusion in the interaction between human and machine could have serious consequences. Cognitive ergonomics in these scenarios focuses on designing systems that support rapid, accurate decision-making, minimize error, and create a fluid, natural interaction between human cognition and technology.

Ultimately, human-computer interaction in cognitive ergonomics is about optimizing the relationship between humans and technology by understanding how the mind processes information and responds to digital systems. It involves crafting designs that support the user's cognitive abilities, ensuring that the technology enhances rather than hinders their performance. This alignment between human cognitive processes and system design is key to creating intuitive, efficient, and user-friendly technological experiences.

2.3 Organizational ergonomics

Organizational ergonomics focuses on optimizing sociotechnical systems, which include organizational structures, policies, and processes. The aim is to enhance overall organizational performance by improving communication, teamwork, and work processes, while ensuring that work practices are aligned with human capabilities and needs. Macroergonomics deals with the analysis, design, and evaluation of work systems. Here, "work" refers to any form of human effort or activity, including recreation and leisure, and "system" refers to sociotechnical systems, which can range from a single individual using a tool to the complexity of a multinational organization

[24]. Conceptually, macroergonomics is seen as a top-down approach, but in practice, it involves a combination of top-down, bottom-up, and middle-out processes for analysis, design, and evaluation [24]. A full macroergonomic effort is most feasible under four conditions. First, when creating a new work system from the ground up, such as when forming a new organization. Second, and more commonly, when a significant change to the work system is already planned, such as upgrading equipment, adopting new technology, or relocating to a new facility. A third opportunity arises when there is a major shift in the organization's goals, scope, or direction. Lastly, macroergonomics is crucial when an organization faces a persistent, costly problem that cannot be resolved through micro-ergonomic efforts or other intervention strategies [24]. Often, a full macroergonomic intervention is not immediately feasible. Instead, the ergonomist or ergonomic team may start by implementing micro-ergonomic improvements that deliver quick, positive results—often referred to as the "picking the low-hanging fruit" strategy. As managers observe these successes, they become more inclined to support broader ergonomic interventions. During this process, the ergonomist can raise the awareness of decision-makers about the broader scope of ergonomics and its potential value to the organization [24].

In essence, macroergonomics moves beyond the confines of individual workstations or task-specific interventions, shifting focus toward an overarching strategy that enhances both human well-being and organizational success. It operates at a level where the design of systems must account for the complex, often fluid, relationships between workers, their tools, their tasks, and the organizational goals they strive to achieve. This broader perspective allows for interventions that are not only sustainable but also resilient, capable of adapting to the ever-evolving nature of work in modern organizations. By doing so, macroergonomics helps to foster workplaces that are not just efficient, but also supportive, engaging, and aligned with long-term organizational goals.

2.3.1 Historical development

The concept of designing sociotechnical systems to improve how humans interact with their environment is not something new in the field of ergonomics. In fact, it's been an integral part of the discipline, ever since ergonomics formally took shape in the late 1940s. In the early years, especially during the first few decades, much of the focus was on optimizing the interface between individuals and their immediate work settings—what we now refer to as micro-ergonomics. Back then, this area of study was initially called "man-machine interface design." However, as the society became more aware of gender sensitivities, the term evolved into "human-machine interface design," a more inclusive and thoughtful descriptor. The focus during that time was about understanding human capabilities and limitations—everything from physical to mental characteristics—and using that knowledge to improve how we designed tools, workspaces, control systems, and physical environments. The ultimate goal was to enhance health, safety, comfort, and productivity, while also reducing the chances of human error through better design. With the arrival of the silicon chip and the rapid growth of computers, the focus of ergonomics shifted. The increased automation in sociotechnical systems opened the door for a new subfield within ergonomics, one centered on software design. This new branch, known as cognitive ergonomics, emerged in the mid-1980s. Although the individual operator remained at the heart of the design process, the emphasis shifted toward understanding how humans think, process information, and how software could be developed to communicate in a way that aligns with human cognitive processes. This shift not only advanced the field but also expanded the number of ergonomic positions available in industries worldwide by around 25% [24].

2.3.2 Key focus areas in organizational ergonomics

2.3.2.1 Work system design

Organizational ergonomics focuses on designing work systems that enhance productivity, efficiency, and employee well-being. This approach involves optimizing workflows, job roles, and task assignments to ensure fair and effective work distribution. Such improvements can help reduce the pressures associated with imbalanced workloads and boost overall productivity.

For instance, in a manufacturing plant, organizational ergonomics may involve restructuring the production line to balance the workload among workers. This reduces bottlenecks and minimizes idle time, not only increasing productivity but also reducing work-related stress. Ultimately, these changes lead to improved quality of work life and enhanced health and job satisfaction for employees.

2.3.2.2 Communication and teamwork

Effective communication and teamwork are fundamental to organizational ergonomics, as they enhance team dynamics and streamline information flow. By fostering collaborative workspaces, incorporating advanced communication tools, and establishing clear protocols, this domain ensures that team members interact smoothly and efficiently. In healthcare, for example, organizational ergonomics might involve redesigning hospital ward layouts to facilitate better communication among doctors, nurses, and support staff. This restructuring not only improves patient care but also reduces errors, reinforcing the importance of seamless communication in high-stakes environments.

2.3.2.3 Shift work and scheduling

Shift work presents unique challenges, especially in industries requiring round-the-clock operations. Organizational ergonomics addresses these issues by designing schedules that minimize fatigue, align with workers' circadian rhythms, and incorporate adequate rest breaks. In the transportation sector, for instance, implementing well-structured shift patterns reduces the risk of driver fatigue, thereby enhancing road safety. By prioritizing the health and well-being of shift workers, these ergonomic interventions contribute to a safer and more effective workplace.

2.3.2.4 Organizational culture and change management

The role of organizational ergonomics extends to shaping workplace culture, promoting safety, innovation, and continuous improvement. Ergonomists work with organizations to introduce ergonomic interventions as part of broader change initiatives. In a corporate setting, this may involve implementing wellness programs that encourage regular breaks and a balanced work-life approach, ultimately reducing stress and fostering a healthier, more productive work environment. These changes create a foundation for sustainable workplace improvement and support a culture of ongoing development.

1. Impact on risk reduction: Organizational ergonomics plays a vital role in risk reduction by optimizing work systems, enhancing communication, and nurturing a safety-oriented culture. By addressing these areas, organizational ergonomics helps minimize errors, improve productivity, and elevate workplace satisfaction. It ensures that the work environment supports not only the physical and cognitive needs of workers but also the social dynamics essential for a healthy, efficient workplace.

2. Workplace design: In office settings, ergonomic design is applied to desks, chairs, monitors, and other equipment to minimize strain and prevent injuries. Adjustable chairs, proper desk height, and strategic monitor placement reduce the risk of repetitive strain injuries, such as carpal tunnel syndrome. In industrial environments, ergonomics focuses on designing tools, equipment, and workflows that mitigate the risk of musculoskeletal disorders like back injuries or tendinitis. Ergonomic solutions might include tools that fit comfortably in the hand or workstation adjustments to prevent awkward postures.

3. Product design: Ergonomics is integral in creating user-friendly consumer products, from smartphones to cars, to maximize safety and comfort. For example, smartphones are designed to fit comfortably in the hand, while kitchen appliances feature accessible controls, making them safer and easier to use.

4. Healthcare and rehabilitation: In healthcare settings, ergonomics improves both patient and provider safety by optimizing medical equipment, hospital bed design, and patient-handling procedures. This approach reduces injury risks and enhances care quality. Rehabilitation programs also integrate ergonomic principles to aid recovery and prevent reinjury.

5. Computer and IT equipment: Ergonomically designed keyboards, mice, and monitors help prevent injuries associated with prolonged computer use, such as eye strain, neck pain, and carpal tunnel syndrome. By addressing the ergonomic needs of computer users, these designs promote comfort and reduce strain over extended work hours.

6. Transportation: In the transportation industry, ergonomic design maximizes driver and passenger comfort and reduces fatigue by focusing on adjustable seating, control placements, and dashboard layouts. This attention to ergonomic detail helps enhance safety and usability.

7. Sports and fitness: Sports equipment like bicycles, treadmills, and weight machines benefit from ergonomic design to improve performance and reduce injury risk. Proper ergonomic features help athletes maintain posture, reduce strain, and boost effectiveness during training or competition.

8. Public spaces and furniture: Ergonomics is essential in designing accessible public spaces, such as schools, airports, and theaters, ensuring comfort for diverse users. Seating in these areas is crafted to provide adequate support during extended periods, promoting an inclusive and accommodating environment.

9. Home environment: In home settings, ergonomics improves the functionality of kitchens, bathrooms, and home offices. For instance, kitchen countertops are designed at optimal heights to prevent strain, and frequently used items are arranged within easy reach. Bathrooms are equipped with slip-resistant surfaces and grab bars for safety, while home office setups use adjustable chairs and monitor stands to support good posture and prevent strain injuries.

3. Ergonomics interventions: Modern approaches and technological advancements

The field of ergonomics has evolved significantly in recent years, especially with the integration of advanced technologies. These developments have enhanced the capacity for precise interventions aimed at improving workplace safety, health, and overall productivity. Ergonomics interventions now leverage tools that not only address traditional ergonomic concerns but also introduce novel ways to monitor, assess, and prevent physical strain and musculoskeletal disorders (MSDs).

For instance, the ISCT (infusion set connector tool) could significantly reduce the force and muscle activity while performing ISC task and improved body posture **Figure 2**. In general, ergonomic interventions, such as the design of new tools, are a practical approach to controlling musculoskeletal risk factors and providing a safe and healthy workplace for nurses [25].

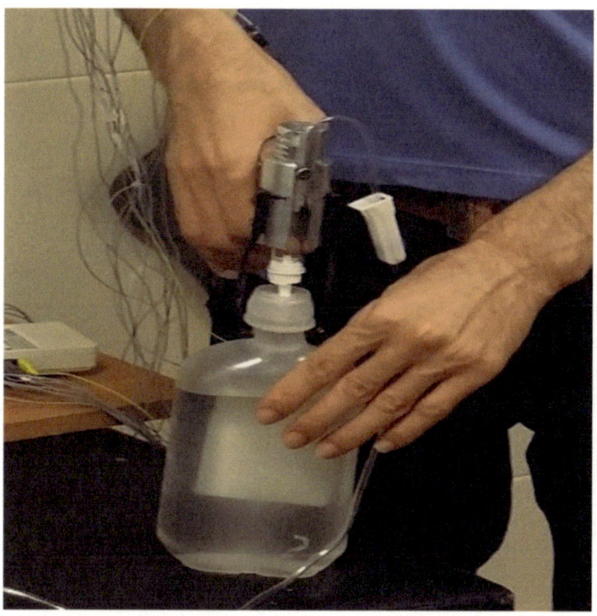

Figure 2.
Infusion set connector tool.

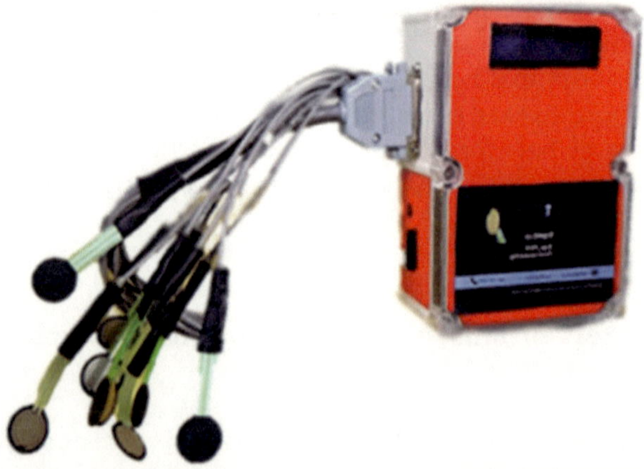

Figure 3.
Example of a device (ErgoFs16) uses Force-Sensitive Resistor (FSR) sensors to measure plantar pressure and detect improper lifting postures in real time.

3.1 Wearable technology for ergonomics monitoring

Recent technological advancements have brought wearable sensors to the forefront of ergonomic interventions. Devices, such as ErgoFs16, as shown in **Figure 3** utilize force-sensitive resistor (FSR) sensors to measure plantar pressure distribution, providing real-time identification of improper lifting postures. By establishing a direct correlation between plantar pressure patterns and ergonomic risk factors, such as UTAH back compressive force and the Lifting Index (LI), it offers a precise and objective method to assess musculoskeletal strain. This capability enhances workplace safety by informing the development of preventive measures and training programs that focus on safe lifting techniques. Additionally, the device's ability to classify lifting postures into safe and hazardous categories supports targeted ergonomic interventions, ultimately reducing the risk of work-related musculoskeletal disorders (WMSDs) [26].

One of the key benefits of wearable technology in ergonomic interventions is the ability to provide real-time feedback to workers. Through mobile apps or connected devices, workers can be alerted to adjust their posture or reduce the intensity of a movement before it results in injury. These technologies are becoming essential in environments where prevention is preferred over post-injury treatment. Additionally, companies are able to aggregate the collected data to identify patterns, allowing for a more holistic approach to reducing workplace injuries by adjusting workflows or providing targeted training sessions.

3.2 Exoskeletons

Another breakthrough in ergonomic intervention is the introduction of exoskeletons, which are wearable devices designed to support the human body during physically demanding tasks. Exoskeletons, both powered and passive, assist workers by redistributing weight, enhancing strength, and reducing fatigue. These devices are particularly beneficial in industries like manufacturing, construction, and healthcare, where manual material handling or repetitive motions often lead to musculoskeletal disorders. Exoskeletons work by alleviating the strain on key areas of the body, such as the lower back, shoulders, and legs. By providing mechanical assistance during lifting or repetitive tasks, they reduce the physical burden on the worker, improving endurance and minimizing the risk of injury. The integration of exoskeletons into ergonomic interventions not only benefits the individual worker by improving comfort and safety but also enhances overall workplace productivity by reducing fatigue and absenteeism.

For instance, the use of the neck exoskeleton was associated with a reduction of muscle electrical activity and the perceived discomfort in the neck area **Figure 4**. These results may be related to transferring neck and head weight by the exoskeleton retaining jack during the neck extension to other areas of the body. The exoskeleton design did not provide support for the shoulder and arm area, which explains the reason for the non-significant results in the shoulder area. Using the exoskeleton with the additional support in shoulder area could be considered as an ergonomic intervention in such overhead works [27].

3.3 Machine learning and predictive modeling in ergonomics

The integration of machine learning algorithms into ergonomics is another pivotal advancement. In conjunction with wearable technologies, machine learning can analyze large datasets collected from workers and predict ergonomic risks. Algorithms, such as Decision Trees (DTs), Support Vector Machines (SVMs), and Random Forests (RFs), are increasingly used to evaluate real-time ergonomic risks by assessing body movements, load handling, and posture deviations. A notable application of this is in manual material handling (MMH), where these models

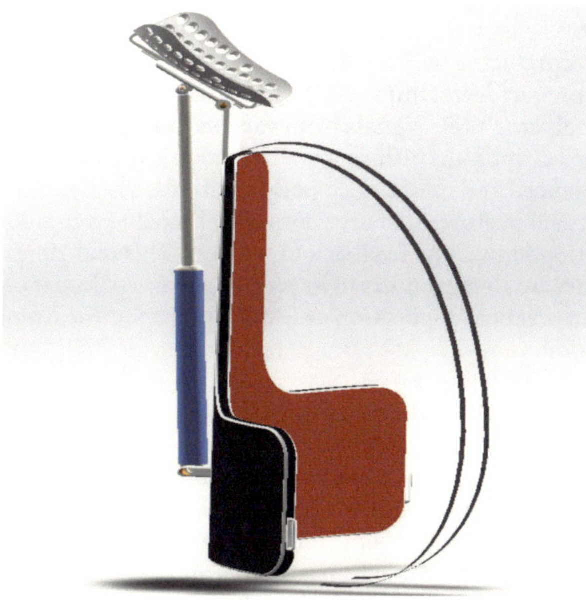

Figure 4.
A scientific innovation—an exoskeleton designed by researchers to support and enhance human strength and endurance in manual tasks. This ergonomic intervention aims to reduce physical strain, prevent musculoskeletal disorders, and improve workplace safety, particularly in industries involving heavy lifting and repetitive movements.

predict the likelihood of musculoskeletal injuries by correlating movement patterns with strain data.

The U.S. National Institute for Occupational Safety and Health (NIOSH) has developed guidelines like the NIOSH Lifting Equation to provide a framework for evaluating ergonomic risks. Recent studies, such as the one using sEMG sensors for ergonomic risk assessment in MMH, have shown that machine learning models can classify risks with high accuracy (close to 99%). These findings mark a significant step forward in automated risk assessment, helping organizations mitigate hazards before they result in injuries, which is especially crucial for workers handling physically demanding tasks.

In a recent research conducted by Varmazyar, M, machine learning techniques are being utilized to identify improper lifting patterns. This approach helps in analyzing the relationship between plantar pressure distribution patterns and the force exerted on the lower back, enabling the design of smart tools like predictive shoes that can alert users during non-ergonomic lifting positions. Such studies highlight the application of machine learning in ergonomics as an innovative method for preventing musculoskeletal disorders.

Machine learning has also been applied in conjunction with surface electromyogram (sEMG)-based systems to enhance ergonomic assessments in manual material handling. In this study, four machine learning models—Decision Tree, Support Vector Machine, K-Nearest Neighbor, and Random Forest—were developed to classify ergonomic risk assessments calculated based on the NIOSH lifting equation. This equation uses a Recommended Weight Limit and Lifting Index to evaluate risk levels in material handling. The study demonstrated that Decision Tree models achieved an accuracy of nearly 99.35% in predicting risk levels, underscoring the potential of machine learning and EMG-based systems for real-time risk detection in tasks that involve lifting and carrying. This approach exemplifies the growing role of machine learning in objectively assessing and mitigating ergonomic risks [28].

A recent study conducted by Sheikh, F utilized both electromyography (EMG) and machine learning to detect improper postures, both symmetric and asymmetric, in real time. By analyzing EMG signals from various muscle groups during different postures, machine learning algorithms were trained to recognize the patterns associated with both balanced and unbalanced body positions. The system was able to identify asymmetrical postures that are commonly linked to musculoskeletal strain and injuries, offering immediate feedback to workers. This real-time detection system helps prevent injury by alerting users to improper posture before it causes harm, demonstrating the practical application of EMG and machine learning in ergonomics for injury prevention.

3.4 Internet of things (IoT) and connected workspaces

The advent of the Internet of Things (IoT) has revolutionized workplace ergonomics. IoT platforms enable the seamless integration of various sensors and devices to create a connected environment where workers' ergonomic health is continuously monitored. For instance, IoT-enabled smart chairs and desks can automatically adjust their height, tilt, or angle to suit individual workers based on real-time feedback. These automated adjustments reduce the strain on workers by promoting healthier postures throughout the day.

In high-risk industries, such as construction, IoT-based systems track vibration exposure, awkward postures, and forceful exertions, which are common precursors to MSDs. The ability to monitor and respond to these risks in real time makes IoT an invaluable tool in preventing ergonomic injuries. Not only does this technology help improve individual worker's health, but it also provides organizational leaders with comprehensive data to develop and refine ergonomics policies.

3.5 Virtual reality (VR) for ergonomic training

Another promising intervention in ergonomics is the use of virtual reality (VR) to simulate workplace environments for training purposes. VR systems allow workers to practice safe lifting techniques, posture corrections, and proper workstation setups in a controlled, immersive environment. This type of intervention is particularly beneficial for training employees in high-risk sectors, such as healthcare, warehousing, and construction, where hands-on experience with ergonomic best practices can significantly reduce injury rates.

By incorporating VR, companies can offer scalable, consistent training programs that ensure employees are aware of ergonomic risks and equipped with the knowledge to mitigate them. Moreover, VR-based ergonomic interventions allow for customizable training scenarios, offering a personalized approach to worker safety and health.

3.6 Advanced robotics and automation

Ergonomics interventions are also increasingly intersecting with robotics. Automated systems and collaborative robots (cobots) are being designed to assist in physically demanding tasks, reducing the need for workers to perform high-risk manual labor. These robots are particularly useful in industries such as automotive manufacturing, where heavy lifting, repetitive tasks, and precision are required. By automating tasks that involve awkward postures, forceful exertions, or repetitive motions, robotic systems help in minimizing the risk of MSDs.

Cobots, in particular, are designed to work alongside human workers, supporting them in lifting heavy materials, assembling parts, or performing repetitive movements that are prone to cause strain. These devices are programmed to operate within safe ergonomic limits, further ensuring the health and safety of workers. The continuous refinement of these robotic systems has led to their increased adoption, allowing organizations to improve both worker safety and operational efficiency.

3.6.1 Conclusion

The latest advancements in ergonomics technology, such as wearable sensors, machine learning models, IoT platforms, VR training, and robotics, have significantly expanded the scope of ergonomic interventions. These technologies are now at the forefront of mitigating workplace risks and preventing musculoskeletal injuries. By incorporating these tools into workplace safety protocols, organizations can not only improve the well-being of their workers but also boost productivity, reduce absenteeism, and minimize compensation costs. The future of ergonomics lies in the continued refinement and integration of these innovative technologies to create safer, more efficient work environments across various industries.

4. Discussion

4.1 Comparisons with recent literature

The findings in this study align with recent advancements in ergonomic interventions using wearable technology. For example, the implementation of sEMG sensors in real-time posture monitoring has been demonstrated to improve risk assessment accuracy, particularly in high-demand industries like manufacturing and construction. Compared to traditional observational methods, wearable devices enable a more granular analysis of muscle strain and movement patterns, making them a valuable asset in managing musculoskeletal disorders (MSDs) associated with manual material handling tasks.

Furthermore, machine learning applications in ergonomic monitoring have advanced significantly, allowing for rapid classification of risk levels and predictive modeling of injury probability. These developments are reflected in studies where models like Support Vector Machines (SVMs) and Decision Trees (DTs) have been used to enhance the prediction accuracy for unsafe postures, supporting a shift from reactive to preventive occupational health measures.

4.2 Global ergonomic practices

Globally, ergonomic practices across various industries are increasingly integrating technologies like exoskeletons and Internet of Things (IoT) platforms to enhance workforce health and safety. For example, automotive companies such as Hyundai employ exoskeletons to support assembly line workers in tasks like undercarriage assembly, where the physical strain is high. Similarly, in the United States, IBM uses IoT-enabled ergonomic systems within their office environments to monitor and dynamically adjust workstation setups based on employees' posture and movement patterns, promoting healthier work habits and reducing strain over time.

These examples illustrate how diverse industries—ranging from manufacturing to corporate office settings—leverage wearable technologies and IoT to create adaptive ergonomic solutions. By providing real-time data on body posture, motion, and force exertion, these systems enable on-the-spot ergonomic adjustments that contribute to long-term workforce well-being. Such implementations demonstrate that advanced technology integration into ergonomics can significantly reduce the risk of work-related musculoskeletal disorders (MSDs) and associated health costs, making workplaces safer and more sustainable across various sectors.

4.3 Limitations

Several limitations emerged in this study that may impact the generalizability of the findings. First, the sample size, though sufficient for initial assessments, limits broader applicability, particularly in a diverse workforce with varying ergonomic needs. Additionally, the use of sEMG sensors, while highly effective, may be constrained by factors like sensor displacement during strenuous tasks, which could affect signal accuracy and data integrity.

The lack of data from certain occupational settings, such as healthcare or warehousing, further limits the scope of this study. Expanding research to include these diverse environments would help validate the current findings and enhance their applicability.

4.4 Suggestions for future research

Future studies should explore a broader range of ergonomic sensors beyond sEMG, such as gyroscopic sensors or pressure mats, which could provide a more comprehensive understanding of body mechanics under varying loads. Additionally, applying deep learning models like Long Short-Term Memory (LSTM) networks may improve classification accuracy for real-time posture detection, especially in dynamic tasks where multiple postures are required.

Furthermore, collaborative studies examining the effectiveness of mixed technologies—such as combining IoT, VR training, and machine learning—could deepen insights into ergonomic interventions, allowing organizations to implement holistic solutions that cover both physical and cognitive ergonomics.

4.5 Key findings and practical implications

This study highlights the effectiveness of using sEMG sensors combined with machine learning models for comprehensive ergonomic risk assessments. By enabling real-time feedback to workers and management, these technologies support proactive interventions that help prevent MSDs, improve productivity, and create safer work environments. The findings suggest significant potential for industries with high ergonomic risk factors, such as construction, healthcare, and manufacturing, where precise posture monitoring and reduction of physical strain are essential for maintaining worker's health.

To expand on these insights, it is recommended that organizations adopt advanced AI-driven technologies, including machine learning, for more sophisticated identification, evaluation, and control of ergonomic risks. Leveraging these technologies can enhance ergonomic interventions by providing continuous, precise assessments of workplace conditions, thereby allowing for more effective, data-driven risk mitigation strategies. These advancements in AI-based ergonomic solutions can reduce injury rates, enhance workforce well-being, and ultimately promote a more resilient and sustainable work environment across various sectors.

4.6 Conclusion

This chapter highlights the critical role of ergonomic interventions in minimizing workplace risk, particularly for musculoskeletal disorders (MSDs). Modern ergonomic approaches leveraging wearable technology, VR, and IoT offer innovative solutions that support both physical and cognitive aspects of ergonomics. For practitioners and policymakers, these findings underscore the importance of integrating these advanced interventions into occupational health strategies to enhance employee well-being and productivity. By focusing on adaptable and data-driven interventions, future ergonomic practices can further align with evolving workplace needs and improve risk management outcomes.

Acknowledgements

The author acknowledges the use of GPT-4, an AI developed by OpenAI, for language polishing of the manuscript.

Author details

Ehsan Garosi*, Fatemeh Sheikh and Mahsa Goodarzi
Iran University of Medical Sciences, Iran

*Address all correspondence to: e-garosi@alumnus.tums.ac.ir

References

[1] Bridger R. Introduction to Human Factors and Ergonomics. Boca Raton: CRC Press; 2017

[2] Wickens CD, Helton WS, Hollands JG, Banbury S. Engineering Psychology and Human Performance. New York: Routledge; 2021

[3] Branaghan RJ, Lafko S. Cognitive ergonomics. In: Clinical Engineering Handbook. Amsterdam, Netherlands: Elsevier; 2020. pp. 847-851

[4] Baddeley AD, Hitch GJ. Developments in the concept of working memory. Neuropsychology. 1994;**8**(4):485

[5] Baddeley A. Working memory: Theories, models, and controversies. Annual Review of Psychology. 2012;**63**(1):1-29

[6] Cowan N. The magical number 4 in short-term memory: A reconsideration of mental storage capacity. Behavioral and Brain Sciences. 2001;**24**:87-185

[7] Ericsson KA, Kintsch W. Long-term working memory. Psychological Review. 1995;**102**(2):211

[8] Sowa JF. Principles of Semantic Networks: Explorations in the Representation of Knowledge. California, USA: Morgan Kaufmann; 2014

[9] Mandler JM. Stories, Scripts, and Scenes: Aspects of Schema Theory. New York, USA: Psychology Press; 2014

[10] Dismukes RK. Prospective memory in workplace and everyday situations. Current Directions in Psychological Science. 2012;**21**(4):215-220

[11] Jolly JD, Hildebrand EA, Branaghan RJ. Better instructions for use to improve reusable medical equipment (RME) sterility. Human Factors. 2013;**55**(2):397-410

[12] Loftus GR. Evaluating forgetting curves. Journal of Experimental Psychology: Learning, Memory, and Cognition. 1985;**11**(2):397

[13] Kieras DE, Bovair S. The role of a mental model in learning to operate a device. Cognitive Science. 1984;**8**(3):255-273

[14] Branaghan RJ, Covas-Smith CM, Jackson KD, Eidman C. Using knowledge structures to redesign an instructor–operator station. Applied Ergonomics. 2011;**42**(6):934-940

[15] Duit R. On the role of analogies and metaphors in learning science. Science Education. 1991;**75**(6):649-672

[16] Nielsen J. Coordinating user interfaces for consistency. ACM Sigchi Bulletin. 1989;**20**(3):63-65

[17] Simon HA. Theories of Bounded Rationality. Amsterdam, Netherlands: North-Holland Publishing Company; 1964

[18] Gigerenzer G, Todd PM. Fast and frugal heuristics: The adaptive toolbox. In: Simple Heuristics That Make us Smart. Oxford, England: Oxford University Press; 1999. pp. 3-34

[19] Longo L, Wickens CD, Hancock G, Hancock PA. Human mental workload: A survey and a novel inclusive definition. Frontiers in Psychology. 2022;**13**:883321

[20] Mitchell DK, Abounader B, Henry S, Animashaun A. A Procedure for Collecting Mental Workload Data during

an Experiment That is Comparable to Imprint Workload Data. Tech Rep ARL-TR2009. Maryland, USA: U.S. Army Research Laboratory (ARL); 2009. p. 5020

[21] Longo L. Human-computer interaction and human mental workload: Assessing cognitive engagement in the World Wide Web. In: Human-Computer Interaction–INTERACT 2011: 13th IFIP TC 13 International Conference, Lisbon, Portugal, September 5-9, 2011, Proceedings, Part IV 13. New York City, USA: Springer; 2011

[22] Longo L. Formalising human mental workload as a non-monotonic concept for adaptive and personalised web-design. In: User Modeling, Adaptation, and Personalization: 20th International Conference, UMAP 2012, Montreal, Canada, July 16-20, 2012, Proceedings 20. Springer; 2012

[23] Cain B. A Review of the Mental Workload Literature. Virginia, USA: DTIC Document; 2007

[24] Hendrick H, Kleiner B. Macroergonomics. Theory, Methods, and Applications. 2002;**2002**:1-409

[25] Garosi E, Mazloumi A, Kalantari R, Vahedi Z, Shirzhiyan Z. Design and ergonomic assessment of an infusion set connector tool used in nursing work. Applied Ergonomics. 2019;**75**:91-98

[26] Mehridiz H, Ghasemi MS, Saeedi H, Varmazyar M, Garosi E. Analyzing the correlation between plantar pressure distribution and UTAH back compressive force and NIOSH lifting index in symmetrical lifting tasks. Journal of Health and Safety at Work. 1 Jan 2024;**14**(2):272-290

[27] Garosi E, Mazloumi A, Jafari AH, Keihani A, Sharifnezhad A, Shamsipour M, et al. The effect of using cervical exoskeleton on the neck and shoulder muscles electrical activity during overhead work. Journal of Health & Safety at Work. 2022;**12**(2):259-273

[28] Mudiyanselage SE, Nguyen PHD, Rajabi MS, Akhavian R. Automated workers' ergonomic risk assessment in manual material handling using sEMG wearable sensors and machine learning. Electronics. 2021;**10**(20):2558

Chapter 5

Occupational Sleep Medicine: The Sleep-Related Breathing Disorders in High-Risk Occupations

Martin Popević

Abstract

Sleep-related breathing disorders, primarily obstructive sleep apnea (OSA), have a major impact on the occurrence of excessive daytime sleepiness, sleepiness behind the wheel, and on the occurrence of traffic accidents. It is estimated that almost one billion people worldwide have OSA, while 425 million people suffer from a moderate and severe form of this disease, but that the disease is not recognized in 85% of patients. Drivers with untreated or undiagnosed OSA are two to seven times more likely to be involved in a traffic accident. People working in high-risk occupations, especially safety sensitive jobs, such as commercial drivers, heavy machinery operators, railroad workers, airline pilots, and military personnel, are the most vulnerable category due to significant risk to personal and public safety and health. Despite mandatory medical screening, OSA prevalence in these occupational groups is estimated to be 26–70%, leading to accidents and injuries on and off work, with high costs to employees, employers, and society in general. Further measures should be taken in adequate education, screening, diagnostic, and treatment procedures in order to reduce the burden of sleep-related breathing disorders and its consequences in high-risk professions.

Keywords: sleep apnea, excessive sleepiness, high-risk occupations, commercial drivers, traffic accidents

1. Introduction

1.1 Sleep

Sleep is defined as a reversible behavioral state of perceptual exclusion from the environment and a state of relative insensitivity to events in the environment, which has specific behavioral characteristics, such as physical rest, stereotyped position, and specific sleeping place. Sleep is characterized by an elevated threshold for awakening and reactivation but also rapid awakening after intense stimulation, as well as specific changes in biological processes (breathing, heartbeat, hormone secretion, and thermoregulation). One of the physiological characteristics of sleep is the need to compensate for sleep in case of deprivation [1].

It is much more difficult to define what normal sleep is. Buysse et al. [2] believe that the most important elements of healthy sleep are duration, efficiency, sleep schedule, daytime alertness, and sleep quality.

Sleep disorders are very common in the general population. Morin et al. state that 8–18.5% of the adult population are not satisfied with the quality or quantity of their sleep, and that 10% of respondents consider that they have bad sleep [3]. In a large survey [4] in a representative sample of US citizens (The National Health and Nutrition Examination Survey, NHANES), as many as one-third of respondents stated that they had poor sleep (34.3–35.2%). This problem is even more pronounced in the elderly population, where it is believed that as many as 50% of people have problems initiating or maintaining sleep [5].

The current research recognizes the strong association of sleep disorders, especially obstructive sleep apnea, with excessive daytime sleepiness, accidents and injuries at work, traffic accidents, as well as cardiovascular, respiratory, metabolic, neurological, psychiatric, and malignant diseases.

Therefore, the recognized influence of sleep-related disorders on work ability and quality of life in the adult population soon became of interest in the health and safety community. The job-related risks of sleep disorders are significantly higher in people working in high-risk occupations, such as commercial drivers, train operators, airline pilots, and first responders, so there is a growing need for preventive measures by the employers, employees, health, and safety experts as well as community in general.

1.2 Stages of sleep

Sleep in its essence is not a state, but a multi-phase essential process with cyclic repetitions at certain time intervals. With the discovery and application of electroencephalography (EEG), and later with the addition of electrooculography (EOG), electromyography (EMG) and electrocardiography (ECG), it was established that two basic stages can be defined during sleep, designated as REM ("Rapid Eye Movement") and NREM (non-REM).

In physiological conditions, NREM constitutes the largest part of sleep, with the dominance of homeostatic mechanisms of the body's vital functions (breathing, heartbeat, hormone secretion, and thermoregulation). Breathing slows down, the tidal volume decreases, and the sensitivity of chemoreceptors to CO_2 and O_2 decreases, with an increase in the partial pressure of CO_2. Due to the predominance of parasympathetic control of the autonomic nervous system, the heartbeat slows down. NREM contains three sub-stages (N1, N2, and N3).

The waking state is characterized by low-voltage EEG activity of a variable frequency range, often associated with high muscle tone and fast eyeball movements (blinking, reading, and viewing movements). When falling asleep or closing the eyes, the so-called alpha activity (frequencies 8–13 Hz) begins to dominate in the EEG of most people. The N1 phase essentially represents the transitional phase from wakefulness to sleep and is characterized by a slowing of the EEG frequency (4-7 Hz), slow rolling movements of the eyeballs, and a relatively lower muscle tone compared to wakefulness. When a person enters the N2 stage, they are considered to be no longer aware of their surroundings. EEG activity is still low-voltage, frequencies 4–7 Hz, but characteristic changes occur in the form of sleep spindles and K complexes. The N3 stage of sleep is usually referred to as "deep sleep," with a predominance of slow-wave (0.5-2 Hz) high-voltage EEG changes.

In the REM phase of sleep, the instability and variability of the body's vital functions (heart, lungs, and thermoregulation) is expressed, as well as the relative atony of all muscles (except the diaphragm). This stage is often referred to as the "dreaming" stage. The EEG activity is very similar to the activity in the awake and N1 states.

The normal sleep cycle of adults lasts 90–110 minutes, begins with the N1, ends with the REM, and repeats itself 3–6 times during the night. The initial cycles during the night contain more NREM, and later during the night, the duration of REM sleep phases gradually increases (the so-called normal sleep architecture).

In a healthy adult aged 20–30 years, the N1 phase accounts for 2–5%, N2 45–55%, N3 13–23%, and the REM phase 20–25% of the total sleep time. The architecture of sleep changes under physiological conditions with the maturation of the central nervous system and with age. With the aging of a person, the total sleep time, sleep efficiency generally shortens, superficial sleep phases (N1 and N2) are more prevalent in time, as well as the relative stability of REM duration [6].

1.3 Regulation of ventilation in the wake/sleep cycle

Control of breathing relies to a large extent on several groups of neurons with inspiratory or expiratory activity, located in the pontomedullary part of the brain stem. The basic generators of the respiratory rhythm are neurons in the ventral respiratory column (VRC), the dorsal respiratory group (DRG) of the nucleus of the solitary tract (*n. tractus solitarii,* NTS), and the pontine ventral group. These neurons are influenced by information from higher regions of the cerebrum. The ventrolateral part of the medulla oblongata is the central location of respiratory neurons, where the main generator of inspiratory activity is the so-called pre-Botzinger complex, and the regulator of expiratory activity and the normal breathing cycle is the Botzinger complex. In addition to the above, the role in regulation is played by the retrotrapezoid nucleus (RTN, chemosensitivity during wakefulness). Information to the respiratory centers comes from peripheral chemoreceptors, baroreceptors, respiratory muscles, and stretch receptors in the lungs via vagal afferent fibers to the NTS and, after multilevel processing and integration, to the respiratory centers. The feedback of breathing regulation includes the modulation of the activity of the muscles involved in the breathing process, at rest, during effort, and during large metabolic variations. The cerebral cortex influences breathing during the voluntary activities of speech and swallowing.

Normal breathing is generally not registered consciously; however, any indication of difficulty breathing (physical effort, stressful situation, and lack of air) triggers a complex cascade of reactions of the central nervous system in order to maintain the vital function of the organism [6].

The respiratory center located in the medulla oblongata and pons receives and responds to chemical (oxygen, carbon dioxide, and hydrogen ions) and mechanical stimuli (stretching of the lungs and chest wall), as well as to behavioral information. The partial pressure of O_2 is detected via receptors in the carotid and aortic bodies, and the information is transmitted to the brain via the fibers of the glossopharyngeal nerve. The partial pressure of CO_2 is registered through receptors in the carotid body and through the central medullary chemoreceptor. An increase in pCO_2 and hydrogen ions directly stimulate the respiratory center, leading to an increase in ventilation, unlike pO2, which has a positive effect on ventilation only if it falls below 7.3 kPa.

In addition to the chemical control of breathing, the mechanical load of the respiratory system, through the stretching of the receptors in the lung tissue, leads to an increase in impulses to the medulla oblongata via the vagus nerve. In the awake state, metabolic control mechanisms can be modified voluntarily. The respiratory center sends feedback signals to the respiratory muscles. During breathing, signals sent to the muscles of the upper respiratory tract lead to a decrease in compliance and the possibility of pharyngeal collapse at negative intrapleural pressure [6].

During sleep, ventilation is dominantly dependent on metabolic control mechanisms, with the main stimulus being the partial pressure of CO_2 in the arterial blood. In physiological conditions, there is a decrease in the ventilatory response to hypercapnia and hypoxemia, with the appearance of hypoventilation, CO_2 retention, increased resistance in the airways, decreased reflexes, and occasional apneas when the mechanical load increases. There is also a decrease in impulses from the medullary inspiratory cells to the phrenic and hypoglossal nerves, with a decrease in the work of the thoracic pump and an increase in resistance in the upper airways. Central sensitivity to chemical stimuli also decreases, leading to CO_2 retention, and additionally lower reactions to variations of O_2 and CO_2 in the body. On the other hand, hypocapnia during hyperventilation easily leads to central apneas and also reduces motor impulses to the respiratory muscles, facilitating the occurrence of obstructive respiratory events. Sympathetic vasoconstriction is also reduced during sleep, which may contribute to pharyngeal narrowing via vasodilation and tissue edema.

The aforementioned disorders become even more pronounced with the entry into the REM phase of sleep, when the tone of the striated muscles further deteriorates, the dependence of breathing on the activity of the diaphragm increases, and the response to chemical stimuli decreases [6, 7].

1.4 Sleep disorders

According to the International classification of sleep disorders (ICSD-3rd revision) [8], there are several categories of sleep disorders, ranging from insomnia, sleep-related breathing disorders, central disorders of hypersomnolence to circadian rhythm disorders, parasomnias, and sleep-related movement disorders.

1.4.1 Insomnia

Insomnia occurs due to disturbances in the regulation of the wakefulness-sleep cycle and is manifested by insufficient quantity, continuity or quality of sleep, accompanied by cognitive disorders of varying degrees. The prevalence of the disease is in the range of 6–33% of the population, depending on the definition [8, 9].

1.4.2 Narcolepsy

Narcolepsy is a disease caused by a disorder of hypocretin secretion and regulation of the wake-sleep cycle, of still unclear etiology, with the consequent occurrence of pronounced excessive sleepiness, cataplexy, and other REM sleep phenomena such as hypnagogic hallucinations and sleep paralysis. The estimated prevalence of the disease is 25–50 per 100,000, and the incidence is 0.74 per 100,000 person-years [8, 9].

1.4.3 Idiopathic hypersomnia

Idiopathic hypersomnia is a disease of central nervous system origin characterized by normal or extended duration of night sleep, with excessive daytime sleepiness and secondary daytime episodes of NREM sleep, typically lasting 1–2 hours. The estimated prevalence and incidence is 10 to 20 times lower than that of narcolepsy. The disease develops gradually, equally in both sexes, with the first manifestations in the period of adolescence [8, 9].

1.4.4 Circadian rhythm disorders

The main problem in this group of diseases is the incompatibility of the endogenous circadian rhythm of a person and the exogenous rhythm imposed by the social environment (shift work and change of time zones). As a result, during the waking state, the person gets pronounced drowsiness and the need to sleep, and vice versa, during sleep, the person cannot fall asleep. Chronic sleep deprivation progressively increases excessive daytime sleepiness. A disturbed circadian process disrupts the homeostatic process of regulating wakefulness and sleep, so sleep becomes superficial, fragmented, and does not bring recovery. Delayed sleep phase occurs in 0.15% of the population and is manifested by insomnia at the beginning of sleep, that is, the inability to wake up at the desired time [8, 9].

2. Sleep-related breathing disorders

The main feature of this group of disorders is abnormal breathing pattern during sleep, and in some instances, this pattern can be present even after waking up. The most common is obstructive sleep apnea (OSA), followed by central sleep apnea disorders, sleep-related hypoventilation disorders, and sleep-related hypoxemia disorder.

The central sleep apnea (CSA) disorders are recognized by reduction or complete cessation of airflow with low or no respiratory effort due to transient inhibition of ventilatory motor output during sleep. Most of the CSA events are usually seen in NREM sleep [8].

There are several pathophysiological subtypes of CSA, such as high loop gain/increased controller gain CSA (seen in patients with heart failure, atrial fibrillation, acromegaly, chronic renal failure, drug-induced CSA, treatment emergent CSA, high altitude CSA, primary (idiopathic) CSA). Other type is high loop gain/increased plant gain CSA followed by chronic hypercapnia (alveolar hypoventilation, brainstem and spinal cord disorders, neuromuscular disorders, myasthenia gravis, and peripheral nerve disorders). The third type is characterized by the failure of breathing rhythm generation (drug induced-opioid, valproic acid, amyotrophic lateral sclerosis, Parkinson disease, and brainstem disorders).

Some level of CSA can often be seen in patients with OSA, especially in the case of so-called treatment emergent CSA (TECSA), where application of OSA treatment uncovers temporary or permanent central respiratory instability [10].

CSA in patients with congestive heart failure (CHF) often follows the so called Cheyne-Stokes breathing pattern, cyclical crescendo-decrescendo respiration separated by central apneas or central hypopneas. This form of CSA can be seen in male patients over 60 years, in 25–50% of CHF patients, and even 70% of post-stroke patients.

The prevalence of CSA is low in general population. It is estimated that about 4% of patients referred to sleep clinics have some form of central breathing difficulties. CSA is presumed to be present in 10% of people with acromegaly, while almost half of subjects with pulmonary hypertension can present with this type of sleep-related breathing disorder. High altitude CSA can be seen in some healthy individuals at altitudes above 2000 m, with 100% having breathing difficulties at altitudes above 4000 m. Drug-induced CSA can be found in almost one-third of the patients on methadone therapy for heroin addiction [11].

Sleep-related hypoventilation disorders are characterized by an abnormal increase in the arterial PCO2 (PaCO2) during sleep or sleep and wakefulness. The most common are obesity-related hypoventilation syndromes combined with OSA, ranging from obesity-associated sleep hypoventilation, with intermittent or sustained hypercapnia during sleep to full obesity hypoventilation syndrome (hypoventilation during wakefulness, obesity with BMI > 30, not caused by lung or airway diseases). Less common are congenital, idiopathic, and drug or medical disorder-related hypoventilation syndromes [8, 10, 11].

2.1 Obstructive sleep apnea

Obstructive sleep apnea is the most common disorder in the spectrum of sleep breathing disorders and represents a chronic progressive disease with characteristic repetitive interruptions in ventilation during sleep due to complete or partial collapse of the pharyngeal part of the airway. This cessation of breathing is followed by a drop in oxyhemoglobin oxygen saturation and/or awakening [8].

The disorder is clinically defined as the development of characteristic symptoms and signs (excessive daytime sleepiness, loud snoring, recognized interruptions in breathing during sleep or awakening) in the presence of at least five obstructive respiratory events (apnea, hypopnea, or awakenings related to respiratory effort) per hour of sleep. If the number of respiratory events is greater than 15 per hour of sleep, the diagnosis of obstructive sleep apnea can be established independently of the presence and intensity of symptoms. The severity of the disease is predominantly determined based on the number and characteristics of obstructive respiratory events in sleep, through the so-called Apnea-Hypopnea Index (AHI). This index represents the number of objectively registered complete (apnea) or partial (hypopnea) interruptions in breathing per hour of sleep. If the AHI is 5–15 per hour of sleep, a mild to moderate form of OSA is present, if the AHI is 15–30/h moderate to severe, and over 30/h, a very severe form of OSA. The clinical picture, the level, and length of oxyhemoglobin desaturation, the sleep structure disorder and the presence of accompanying diseases are also taken into account [12].

The definition of obstructive sleep apnea continues to evolve in accordance with new knowledge about the etiology, pathogenesis, and consequences of OSA. Two basic questions that arise are the correctness of the definition of respiratory events during sleep (apneas, hypopneas, and awakenings related to respiratory effort) and whether the AHI is a good enough indicator to quantify the severity of the disease. Several indicators have been suggested, such as hypoxic burden, arousal intensity, and cardiopulmonary coupling, but AHI is still in use, as a better indicator of OSA has not yet been found, and the discussion is still ongoing [13–16].

2.1.1 Epidemiology of obstructive sleep apnea

Obstructive sleep apnea is a chronic progressive disease with a high incidence and prevalence in the general population, which without adequate diagnosis and therapy can lead to significant consequences for the health and quality of life of patients [17]. According to the results of large epidemiological studies conducted in Europe, Asia, America, and Australia, about 20% of the adult population has a mild to moderate form of OSA, and 6–7% have a severe and very severe form of OSA. In the studies conducted in the USA, an increase in the prevalence of OSA in the adult population was found, and it is now estimated that about 13% of men and 6% of women aged 30–70 years suffer from a moderate to severe form of the disease [18].

The more recent data for Europe come from research conducted from 2009 to 2013 on a sample of 2121 residents of Lausanne (the so-called Hypnolaus cohort), both sexes, 40–85 years, with a relatively low average body mass index (BMI). The presence of a moderate to severe form of OSA was confirmed by objective methods in 23.4% of women, and as many as 49.7% of men [19].

Benjafield et al. [20] in 2019 have performed an estimation of OSA distribution and prevalence in 193 countries according to available data, and found that more than 936 million people probably have some level of OSA (AHI ≥5 events/h) with 425 million people as having moderate-severe OSA (AHI ≥15 events/h). The prevalence of mild OSA ranged from 7.8% (Hong Kong) to 77.2% (Malaysia), and for moderate to severe OSA, from 4.8% (Ireland and Israel) to 36.6% (Switzerland).

The estimated incidence of the disease is about 7.5% for the moderate to severe form of the disease and for the mild to moderate form of OSA about 16% at the 5-year level [21].

2.1.2 Pathophysiology of obstructive sleep apnea

OSA is based on partial or complete obstruction of the upper airways during sleep, primarily at the level of the pharynx. The mechanism of obstruction includes the interaction of a number of parameters, such as the anatomical characteristics of the airway itself, the critical closing pressure (Pcrit), lung volume and tracheal retraction, the activity of the muscles responsible for the dilatation of the airway (*m. genioglossus*), redistribution of extracellular fluid, and also instability control of ventilation and arousal threshold [22].

2.1.3 Risk factors for obstructive sleep apnea

Risk factors for OSA are male sex, age, central obesity, large neck circumference, facial structure, snoring, alcohol and cigarette consumption, menopause, and the existence of previous diseases (polycystic ovary syndrome and neurological and neuromuscular disorders).

The global obesity epidemic, now affecting more than 2 billion people worldwide, including children, is the probable cause of such high numbers in OSA prevalence.

Important risk factors include menopause (muscle loss, decrease in tone, and redistribution of fat tissue), smoking (chronic inflammation of the upper respiratory tract, increased resistance to air flow, decreased reactivity of the pharynx, and sleep fragmentation), alcohol consumption (reduction of pharyngeal dilator muscle tone and hypoventilation), or use of drugs (impairment of sleep quantity or quality and muscle tone disorder) [23–25]. Genetic predisposition is also recognized, for example, polymorphism of the LEPR, MMP-9, and GABBR1 genes [26].

2.2 Diagnosis of obstructive sleep apnea

The diagnosis is based on the characteristic history and clinical picture of the disease, as well as on the identification of the consequences and complications of the disease [9, 12, 21, 25].

ICSD-3 [8] defines the diagnostic criteria for OSA in three categories, and the information gathered from the patient should be positive in categories A and B or in category C.

Category A defines the presence of one or more symptoms (sleepiness, insomnia, and fatigue), signs (waking up choking, gasping for air, and snoring experienced by the patient or witnessed by bed partner), and characteristic comorbidities (high blood pressure, coronary artery disease, stroke, congestive heart failure, atrial fibrillation, or type 2 diabetes mellitus, depression etc.). Category B is based on objective polysomnography (PSG) or out of center sleep testing (OCST, home sleep apnea test, and HSAT) showing predominantly obstructive respiratory events with AHI ≥5 events/h. Category C is also based on objective polysomnography (PSG) or out of center sleep testing (OCST) showing predominantly obstructive respiratory events with AHI ≥15 events/h.

2.2.1 Anamnesis

Targeted OSA anamnesis is conducted in case the patient complains of symptoms specific to OSA, in patients who are at high risk of OSA (obesity, cardiovascular, respiratory, and metabolic diseases), but also in subjects employed in high-risk occupations (commercial drivers, pilots, train drivers, construction machine operators, military, ambulance, and firemen personnel) [12]. It is necessary to collect information from the patients and members of their immediate family, spouses, children, roommates, and colleagues.

Nocturnal and daytime complaints are characteristic. During the night, a short time of falling asleep is mentioned. Loud snoring, followed by interruptions in breathing, sometimes suffocation, ending with waking up, a feeling of fear, restlessness, palpitations, sweating, heartburn, dry mouth, nocturia, heart palpitations, severe headaches, and difficulty breathing are also possible.

In the morning, the patients report feeling of fatigue, sleepiness, dry mouth, heartburn, or bloating. There could also be a headache, mood issues, irritability, difficulty in focus or memory, especially during monotonous or new activities, fulfilling work and family obligations [27].

During the day, a dominant, but not always clearly present symptom is excessive daytime sleepiness, which can manifest itself in the form of the need to sleep, but also as fatigue, heaviness in the arms and legs, and mental and physical sluggishness. It can be expressed in situations where there is otherwise a high tendency to fall asleep (after a large meal, lying in bed after work) but also in situations that require a high level of alertness (talking, walking, driving a motor vehicle, managing, or monitoring demanding systems).

Patients mostly mention a gradual, long-term development of complaints, with exacerbations during variations in body weight, acute and exacerbations of chronic diseases, after consuming alcohol and drugs with a sedative effect or when sleeping on the back.

In the personal history, often we identify the presence of conditions and disorders that predispose or are consequences of OSA (craniofacial abnormalities, chronic allergic rhinitis, hypertension, heart failure, arrhythmias, cerebrovascular insult, reflux esophagitis, hypothyroidism, and diabetes mellitus). A family tendency toward OSA is often recognized.

2.2.2 Questionnaires

In clinical practice and research, various questionnaires that patients fill out themselves, as well as diagnostic models that combine the patient's subjective data and objective parameters in order to assess the risk of the presence of OSA, are often used as a replacement or supplement to the anamnesis [28].

The Epworth Sleepiness Scale (ESS), measuring average excessive daytime sleepiness, targeted questions (for specific situational sleepiness), the Pittsburgh Sleep Quality Index (PSQI), or the Functional Outcomes of Sleep Questionnaire (FOSQ) are generally used to assess the effects of sleep disorders. There is a certain degree of correlation between the results of these questionnaires and the presence and severity of OSA, but many patients do not have or deny the manifestations of poor sleep, and in some cases, the questions in the questionnaires do not reflect the definitions of sleep problems of the given target group (racial, religious, cultural, socioeconomic, and gender specificities).

A specific problem is the denial or alleviation of symptoms due to the fear of losing a job or the benefits of a certain workplace (commercial drivers, pilots, train drivers, work at height, night work, etc.) [29].

Berlin questionnaire (BQ) was created for OSA screening in primary health care facilities [30]. The questionnaire contains three categories of questions (snoring and shortness of breath, fatigue and sleepiness, and increased blood pressure and obesity) to which the patients answer themselves. If the answers are positive in two or more categories, the person is considered at high risk for the presence of OSA. The questionnaire has been validated in different groups of subjects, from patients presenting to a general practitioner [30–32], to patients with surgical [33], cardiovascular (resistant hypertension and atrial fibrillation) [34, 35], or sleep disorders [36, 37].

The STOP-BANG diagnostic model was created by anesthesiologists as a simple OSA screening method in order to predict the risk of peri- and postoperative complications in patients scheduled for various surgical interventions [38]. It contains eight yes/no questions, of which the patient answers the first four questions himself (snoring, fatigue, shortness of breath, and increased blood pressure), and the next four are answered by a healthcare professional after examining the patient (BMI, age, neck circumference, and gender). According to the initial model, any person with three or more answers is considered high risk for the presence of OSA, but in later works, the author offered additional subcategories [39]. The STOP-BANG model was validated on samples of surgical patients and also patients with progressive neurological diseases (multiple sclerosis) and sleep disorders [40–43].

Despite the characteristic complaints and the high frequency of OSA and comorbidities, it is believed that 85% of patients with a pronounced clinical picture of the disease will never be diagnosed with OSA [44].

2.2.3 Polysomnography

The gold standard for the diagnosis of obstructive sleep apnea syndrome is an all-night complete polysomnography, the so-called type I polysomnography (PSG), which involves simultaneous all-night recording of several electroencephalographic (EEG), electrooculographic (EOG), electromyographic (EMG), and electrocardiographic (ECG) channels, with monitoring of breathing (through the difference in pressure or temperature of inhaled and exhaled air), arterial blood oxygen saturation (pulse oximetry), movements of the chest and abdomen, and the behavior of the patient (audio and video monitoring, supervision of health personnel) [12].

Given that it is a complicated and demanding procedure for the patient, PSG is performed in specialized health institutions (sleep centers and sleep labs), by specially trained health workers [45].

PSG is also the gold diagnostic standard for other sleep-related breathing disorders and other sleep disorders (narcolepsy, periodic limb movements during sleep, parasomnia, epilepsy during sleep, and secondary insomnia) [46].

In recent years, a less demanding examination, the so-called portable cardiorespiratory polygraphy (type III PSG, HSAT, and OCST), has been recommended for OSA diagnosis. This diagnostic procedure involves monitoring fewer parameters (primarily at the expense of sleep indicators and sleep phases – EEG and EOG) and is suitable for use in patients where there is a strong suspicion of OSA in the absence of significant comorbidities and other sleep disorders [12, 47]. The main advantage is the ease of execution, the possibility for the patient to set up the device himself, the examination is performed in home conditions that correspond to the real characteristics of the patient's sleep, and the record analysis is faster, which means that the patient gets a diagnosis and therapy in a shorter time. The main limitation of the portable method is the impossibility of accurately assessing the duration and architecture of sleep and awakening during sleep, which makes the obtained AHI index (in this case, the so-called RDI i.e. Respiratory Disturbance Index) lower by up to 30% compared to the AHI determined by PSG.

Therefore, in all situations when the result of HSAT is negative, and there is a clinical picture or risk factors, the patient must be referred for a PSG, which significantly increases the time and costs of the examination [48].

The technological advances, including machine learning and artificial intelligence, followed by a strong demand (many patients, limited capacities) for easy to use and fast and precise diagnostics of OSA, have led to many new scientifically confirmed diagnostic modalities, such as automated mandibular movement pattern analysis, or use of high-end commercial wrist watches [49, 50].

The American academy of sleep medicine clinical practice guidelines [51] has recognized the possibility of using peripheral arterial tonometry devices (such as WatchPAT) for home sleep testing of patients with suspected OSA, while other technologies, although scientifically sound, have not been proven on the long run to be accepted in the current guidelines.

Still, the sheer number of undiagnosed patients and disproportional availability of these older and newer technologies, as well as educated healthcare professionals around the world, create the need for adequate screening of patients in high risk of OSA. Comparing the results obtained using standard questionnaires with the PSG or HSAT results determined that most OSA questionnaires and diagnostic models show moderate to high sensitivity, accompanied by low to moderate specificity.

Excessive daytime sleepiness represented by a score on the ESS in most cases correlates poorly with the presence and severity of OSA, with low sensitivity and moderate specificity compared to the diagnostic gold standard [52, 53]. In the general population, the BQ showed a relatively low sensitivity (37.2% for AHI $\geq$ 5, 43% for AHI $\geq$ 15), while the specificity reached 84% for AHI $\geq$ 5. Netzer et al. [30] showed high sensitivity for AHI > 5 (86%) and high specificity for moderate and severe OSA (97%) in primary care patients. However, the sensitivity at AHI > 15 or AHI > 30 was relatively low (54 and 17%).

In the initial evaluation on a sample of surgical patients [38], STOP-BANG showed high sensitivity at all AHI thresholds (83.6–100%) and low specificity (highest 56% at AHI > 5). El-Sayed et al. [53] compared the results of four standard OSA questionnaires (ESS, STOP, STOP-BANG, and BQ) with the findings of the gold standard and observed that the BQ and STOP-BANG showed high sensitivity for all levels of OSA severity followed by low specificity. Similar results were obtained by a comparative analysis of five questionnaires with objective methods in Greece [52].

2.3 Treatment of obstructive sleep apnea

The therapeutic approach to a person with OSA must be multidisciplinary, long-term, and individually adapted to the needs of each patient. There are several basic options in the treatment of patients with OSA.

2.3.1 Continuous positive air pressure (CPAP)

In practice, the treatment of choice for most of the patients is application of continuous air therapy, which is transferred to the upper respiratory tract under increased pressure (compared to atmospheric pressure) via a nasal or oral-nasal mask during sleep increases the intraluminal air pressure and prevents airway collapse underlying the obstruction [54]. In addition, CPAP increases the end-expiratory volume of the lungs, along with pulling the upper respiratory tract, strengthening the wall of the pharynx, and contributes to improving the function of the dilator muscles and reducing the edema of soft tissue structures of the pharynx. Despite the almost immediate positive effects, the long-term efficacy, and low costs, the main challenge of CPAP use is still patient adherence and compliance to treatment, so patients often seek other treatment options [55].

2.3.2 Behavioral therapy

In addition to CPAP, an inseparable part of the treatment of OSA is behavioral therapy, that is, correction of bad eating habits, improvement of the quality and quantity of physical and work activity, reduction of body weight, elimination or large reduction of consumption of alcohol, cigarettes, and psychoactive substances that negatively affect the severity and prognosis of the disease.

2.3.3 Positional therapy

One of the simple methods of treating OSA is the so-called positional therapy, which aims to eliminate sleeping on the back.

2.3.4 Intraoral prosthetic systems

In a certain number of patients, positive effects were achieved by using oral prosthetic systems that function according to the principle of pulling out/preventing the tongue protrusion ("Tongue protrusion devices") or the lower jaw ("Mandibular advancement devices", MAD) during sleep. In this way, tongue protrusion and narrowing of the pharyngeal space are prevented, and the tone of the dilator muscles and the shape of the pharynx are improved [56].

2.3.5 Surgical therapy

There is a large number of surgical interventions of lesser or greater degree of complexity and invasiveness, which can be used in the therapy of OSA. These methods are indicated as first-line therapy only in patients with clear craniofacial deformities or soft tissue abnormalities of the oropharyngeal region (tonsillar hypertrophy, depressed soft palate, and hypertrophied long uvula). According to the location and type of tissue on which they are performed, they can be endonasal (septoplasty and turbinectomy), oropharyngeal (soft tissue – tonsillectomy, shortening/elevation of the soft palate and uvula, preventing tongue prolapse, and reducing the volume of the base of the tongue), maxillomandibular (bone-shifting forward jaw), operations on the hyoid bone and epiglottis, and removal of parapharyngeal fat pads [57, 58].

2.3.6 Other methods

Pharmacological therapy of OSA is based on the modification of ventilation control, sleep structure (by suppressing REM), or increasing the tone of the pharyngeal dilator muscles. Tricyclic antidepressants, serotonin reuptake inhibitors, cholinergic agents, and acetazolamide have been tried in small studies with conflicting results [59].

The latest research shows the positive effects of electrical stimulation of the hypoglossus via electrodes from a subcutaneously implanted system in patients with moderate and severe OSA. Nerve activation increases the tonic and phasic activity *of the genioglossus muscle* and the stability of the pharyngeal part of the airway. Significant reductions in sleepiness, improvement in sleep quality, reduction in AHI, degree and duration of desaturations were registered, and the effects persisted even after 18 months from the start of administration [60].

2.4 Consequences of obstructive sleep apnea

In the event that OSA is not diagnosed on time or treated adequately, the disease progresses and is accompanied by significant health disorders.

The underlying pathophysiological mechanisms of OSA, intermittent hypoxia, and sleep fragmentation are responsible for a wide range of secondary health impairments. OSA is often present in people with micro- and macro-vascular endothelial dysfunction [61], subclinical atherosclerosis [62], and developed cardiovascular disorders (arterial hypertension, heart failure, atrial fibrillation, and ischemic heart disease) and is an independent risk factor for the occurrence of these diseases [63]. It is believed that approximately 50% of patients with arterial hypertension suffer from OSA, and the disease is often associated with a non-dipping pattern of hypertension and an increase in blood pressure in patients with a resistant form of arterial hypertension [64]. There is a clear association between the presence of untreated and severe OSA with an increase in total mortality and mortality from coronary events.

OSA often follows or aggravates chronic obstructive pulmonary disease (so-called Overlap syndrome) and bronchial asthma. There is a clear correlation between the OSA and metabolic disorders, such as insulin resistance, diabetes mellitus, and metabolic syndrome. OSA can often be found in people suffering from depression, gastroesophageal reflux, and other diseases [4, 17, 25]. Patients with untreated OSA have a significantly higher number of intra- and postoperative complications, return to intensive care units more often and stay longer in the hospital compared to patients with treated OSA or patients without OSA [65].

2.5 Drowsiness and obstructive sleep apnea

Excessive daytime sleepiness is one of the main features of OSA and is often the main reason OSA patients see their doctor. Drowsiness occurs in milder forms in situations with a high degree of somnificity (after a meal, lying down, watching television), and in more severe forms, in situations that require a greater degree of alertness (speech, walking, and mentally demanding tasks), significantly impairing the patients' ability to live and work [8]. According to data from the Sleep Heart Health survey [66], excessive sleepiness is reported by 38.5% of subjects with AHI > 5/h, 46% with AHI > 15/h and 51.4% of subjects with AHI > 30/h. In a study of a large sample of OSA patients in Spain [67], the prevalence of self-reported excessive sleepiness was about 57%.

There is a positive but not strong correlation between the OSA severity and the degree of subjectively or objectively assessed sleepiness [68–70]. Research by Roura et al. [67], as well as by Mediano et al. [71], showed that sleepy OSA patients have shorter sleep latencies, longer sleep duration, more slow-wave sleep, and higher sleep efficiency, indicating that the underlying issue may not be sleep deprivation. It is possible that the degree of sleepiness is influenced by the presence of comorbidities (obesity, diabetes, and depression) [69, 72, 73] and the degree of oxidative stress and inflammation caused by intermittent hypoxia [74]. Patients with OSA and cardiovascular disorders complain lack of sleepiness, possibly due to increased activity of the sympathetic system [75, 76].

Subjective and objective sleepiness are also subject to changes with aging. It is believed that in older age, patients attach less importance to sleepiness, mainly due to its lesser impact on their quality of life and work compared to other health problems [77].

Application of basic OSA symptomatic treatment significantly reduces the degree of subjective and objective sleepiness, even in mild forms of the disease [78, 79]. Generally, the symptoms of drowsiness subside faster and more intensively compared to objective indicators, but in a certain number of cases (6%), drowsiness persists despite therapy [80]. The causes of this so-called residual excessive sleepiness are individual, and range from inadequately dosed and applied therapy, through comorbidities, to irreversible central damage to neurons controlling wakefulness and sleep [81].

In addition to excessive sleepiness, 80% of patients with an undiagnosed or untreated form of the disease also have disorders of neurocognitive functions, primarily in the domain of attention, memory, and executive functions [82], and 50% of patients also have personality disorders. Attention is impaired in all three domains – extended, divided, and selective attention, which also contributes to impaired executive functions (mental flexibility, inhibition, short-term memory, and problem solving). The application of CPAP therapy leads to a large degree of improvement, but not to a complete recovery. Motor coordination and reaction speed are impaired, which do not improve with therapy, indicating permanent cortical damage caused by OSA [83]. As a consequence of these damages, there are problems in performing daily activities, including work tasks. There is a decrease in work ability, and on the other hand, there is an increase in the risk of injury at work (relative risk 2.88) and absence from work [84, 85].

2.6 OSA and traffic accidents

One of the cardinal manifestations of OSA, excessive daytime sleepiness has long been recognized as an important cause of traffic accidents. Therefore, it is not surprising that the link between OSA and accidents was established very quickly.

The first descriptions of the syndrome identified patients having drowsiness or falling asleep while driving or developing amnesia for parts of the road traveled in traffic [86].

Young et al. [87] investigated the frequency of traffic accidents in subjects from the general population included in one of the largest natural course studies of sleep-disordered breathing (Wisconsin Sleep Cohort Study). They found that men with AHI > 5 are three times more likely to experience an accident, and that respondents of both sexes with AHI > 15 are seven times more likely to experience multiple accidents in a five-year interval. Excessive daytime sleepiness did not significantly affect the estimated risk of accidents. The first large systematic review on the relationship between OSA and traffic accidents was published in 2006 [88]. The main conclusion was there is a clear association of OSA and traffic accidents, with odds ratio from 1.3 to 13 (average value 3). OSA severity, but not daytime sleepiness correlated with the occurrence of accidents. OSA treatment led to a reduction in traffic accident risk.

A meta study by Sassani et al. [89] found that treating OSA in all diagnosed US drivers would cost $3.18 billion, but would result in savings of $11.1 billion and save 980 lives on an annual basis.

In a meta-analysis published in 2009 [90], Tregear et al. confirmed the fact that drivers suffering from unrecognized or untreated OSA have a two- to three-fold increased risk of being involved in a serious traffic accident compared to drivers without OSA (relative risk 2,43). The main risk factors for accidents in OSA drivers were BMI, AHI, and degree of hypoxemia, while the excessive sleepiness was probably important. In a meta-analysis published in 2010 [91], the same research group showed that the use of CPAP led to a significant reduction in the risk of traffic accidents in OSA patients. The effects of CPAP on sleepiness were noticeable after just 1 day, while improvements in the ability to drive were seen within 2 to 7 days.

In a recent systematic review and meta-analysis [92], the odds of car accidents were found to be more than double in subjects with OSA (OR = 2.36), with a slightly higher risk in commercial drivers (OR = 2.80) compared to amateur drivers (OR = 2.32). No significant correlation was found between sleepiness and car crashes.

3. High risk occupations

High-risk jobs [93] involve tasks and responsibilities that put an individual's physical as well as their mental health to a greater risk level than ordinarily. These jobs tend to require more skills, training, and commitment. High risk may be due to handling of heavy machines (forklifts, cranes, transporters, construction, and agricultural machinery, etc.), truck/bus driving, dealing with toxic substances, working at height/under ground level or working in inadequate work environment (noise, vibration, radiation, and high/low temperature). People working in high risk jobs are usually those that have greater chances of being involved in accidents or injuries. High-risk jobs also often require use of personal protective equipment.

Safety-sensitive jobs [94] are a specific category of high-risk jobs, including positions that place others at risk of injury or hurt in the event of poor performance of related work tasks or activities by an employee. For instance, safety-sensitive jobs include pilots, truck drivers, high competence machine operators, railroad operators, military personnel, first responders (firefighters, paramedics, and police) construction workers, and healthcare workers.

Most of the available literature on sleep related breathing disorders in high risk occupations deals with OSA. The probable reason is that the other disorders, such as CSA, OHS are lower in prevalence, more difficult to diagnose, and often interrelated with OSA. On the other hand, may be we are seeing a form of "healthy worker effect," due to possibility that the subjects who had these types of disorders could not pass the mandatory medical examination for high-risk occupations.

The primary high-risk occupational group are commercial drivers, due to recognized OSA effect on frequency and severity of traffic accidents.

3.1 Commercial drivers

There are two basic definitions of commercial drivers. In a broader sense, any person who drives a motor vehicle as part of their job can be considered a professional driver. These include drivers of light and heavy delivery vehicles and bus and taxi drivers but also ambulance drivers, firefighters, field salesmen, couriers, etc.

In a narrower sense, the definition of a professional driver refers only to persons engaged in the transport of goods and passengers by means of trucks and busses, who must meet certain standards of training and psycho-physical abilities to drive said vehicles [95]. According to US standards, a professional driver is any person who holds an adequate driver's license and drives a commercial motor vehicle, that is, a vehicle for the transport of goods or passengers that weighs more than 4500 kg or is designed to transport more than 16 people or serves to transport hazardous materials [96].

3.1.1 Job characteristics of commercial drivers

Commercial drivers are exposed to a large number of dangers and harms that can lead to health disorders [97–99].

Primary risk is the possibility of traffic accidents injury, while driving, getting in and out of the vehicle, loading and unloading cargo, or working around the vehicle (repairs, attaching or detaching the trailer, etc.). When transporting explosive or flammable material (fuel, gases, etc.), there is a possibility of injury in a fire. We should also not forget the dangers of atmospheric electric discharges when driving during inclement weather.

Recognized physical hazards at the workplace of commercial drivers are exposure to general noise and vibrations, non-ionizing radiation (UV spectrum – work in open space) and ionizing radiation (transporting radioactive material). The most common chemical hazards are related to the load of the vehicle (gases, fuel, and chemicals in tanks), the working environment (mines, smelters, petrochemical industry, and agriculture) or the vehicle itself (motor, brake and hydraulic oils, fuel, and exhaust gases). In the case of transporting biological material (people, animals, meat products, leather, wheat, grain, corn, fertilizer, etc.), there is a possibility of biohazard exposure.

Concerning the psychosocial burdens of the driver's workplace, it is observed that commercial drivers are often engaged in extended, irregular, shift, and night work. Transporting certain cargo or people often requires arriving at the destination within a precise time interval, so a planned break during work is often secondary to the punctuality of the delivery. A significant percentage of commercial drivers is self-employed, with their own vehicles, so the time of work and rest depends on the volume of work and earning potential. Due to long-term work in the field, the problem of irregular and improper nutrition and sleep also arises. Due to prolonged and night work, as well as sleep restriction, drivers face the problem of physiological and pathological sleepiness, and in an attempt to maintain an alert state, they often consume cigarettes, drinks with a high content of caffeine and taurine (energy drinks), as well as carbohydrate-rich foods.

Ergonomic risks are also very pronounced. Commercial drivers spend most of their working time in a sitting position, with a fixed position of the lower and upper extremities, and a smaller part of their working time is spent in physically demanding activities in forced positions (bent, squatting, working with hands above the head, etc.). There is also vision strain due to driving in conditions of reduced visibility. A specific problem is violence at the workplace, conflicts with business associates, colleagues, bosses, and passengers.

3.1.2 Drowsiness and traffic accidents of commercial drivers

Factors that contribute to sleepiness in commercial drivers are identical to factors in the general population and amateur drivers (sleep deprivation and fragmentation, effects of circadian rhythms, driving time, monotony, and individual characteristics). Prolonged, shift, and irregular work significantly prolongs the awake state and disturbs and shortens the time spent in sleep. In addition, working at night and starting to drive in the early morning is strongly influenced by circadian rhythms and the need for sleep, while daytime sleep after that does not represent an adequate replacement in either quantity or quality of sleep. Unlike amateur drivers, commercial drivers actively participate in traffic 8–16 hours a day, which requires high focus and drains the body's protective mechanisms, leading to fatigue, and drowsiness. The transport of goods and people in good part involves driving on large regional roads and highways, at a controlled speed, with few breaks, with the consequent monotony and feeling of boredom of the driver. In addition, the irregularity of diet, physical activity, and sleep, as well as reduced accessibility of preventive and curative health care influence the occurrence of excessive sleepiness [100].

In an anonymous 2012 National Sleep Foundation survey of employees in all U.S. transportation sectors, 55–60% of truck and bus drivers report getting less than 7 hours of sleep on a weekday [101]. Hanowski et al. study found average sleep time of 6 hours in a 24-hour period, with shorter sleep duration the night before an accident [102]. The National Transportation Safety Board (NTSB) in the USA determined that 52% of accidents involving one truck were associated with sleep disorders and in 18% of cases the drivers admitted to falling asleep while driving [103].

In a large number of countries, legislation has been adopted to regulate the working, driving and rest time for commercial drivers. For example, in the countries of the European Union, EU directive no. 561/2006 [104] is in force, according to which the daily driving period must not exceed 9 hours, except twice a week, when it can be 10 hours. A break of at least 45 minutes (or two breaks of 15 + 30 minutes) must be taken every 4.5 hours of driving. Weekly driving time must not exceed 56 hours, and biweekly driving time must not exceed 90 hours. Rest time during the day must be at least 11 hours, but it can be 9 hours three times a week. Daily rest can be in two parts of a total duration of 12 hours (9 + 3 hours). On a weekly basis, there must be a rest period of at least 45 continuous hours, no longer than every 6 days, except for bus drivers operating international tours where it can be for 12 days. In addition to these basic rules, each EU member state can set additional restrictions or reliefs for certain branches of industry.

4. OSA and commercial drivers

Research conducted worldwide indicates that the prevalence of OSA in the population of commercial drivers is in the range of 20–80%. This discrepancy stems from differences in the definition of OSA, the method of confirming the diagnosis, but also the characteristics of the sample (age, ethnic composition, way of working, type of vehicle, etc.).

A significant number of studies were based on OSA risk assessment questionnaires, primarily BQ, due to objective obstacles related to the organization of stationary tests or examinations in the conditions of bus or truck depots. Moreno et al. [105] investigated the risk of OSA in over 10,000 commercial drivers and found 26% to be at high risk. Amra et al. [106] in an analysis of almost 1000 drivers in Iran found a prevalence of OSA risk of 12.4%, while a study in Malaysia [107] (361) showed about 14.6% of truckers with a positive BQ. In our study [108], BQ recognized 35% subjects as OSA high risk and showed sensitivity of 50.9 (AHI > 5/h) to 75% (AHI > 3/h0), while specificity was 86–70.4% in comparison to PSG or HSAT.

The STOP-BANG diagnostic model has long been used for OSA risk detection in commercial drivers [109].

Ozder et al. [110] found a STOP-BANG score greater than 3 in as many as 71.5% of over 600 bus drivers, and in a similar analysis in Lagos (362) about 50% of respondents were at risk. Our study group identified 69% of commercial drivers' sample as OSA high risk using the same STOP-BANG>3 criteria [111].

In one of the first large studies objectively confirming the presence of OSA in commercial drivers, Stoohs et al. [112] found 78% of the sample of truck drivers from single company had OSA (ODI ≥ 5), and 10% had severe OSA (ODI ≥ 30), associated with the obesity and hypertension. Howard et al. [113] in a two-phase study in Australia, found OSA in almost 60% of drivers, of which 35% mild, 14% moderate, and 10% severe form of the disease. Only 16% of OSA drivers reported sleepiness at the same time. In a recent study, nearly 64% of drivers engaged in public transportation in Taiwan had some form of OSA [114].

In 2006, Alan Pack et al. [115], after a detailed examination of a group of commercial drivers, found that OSA (confirmed by type I PSG) was present in mild form in 17.7%, moderate in 5.8%, and severe form in 4.7% of respondents. In a 2012 study [116], OSA was detected in 43% of truck drivers in Australia. In more recent studies, Karimi et al. [117] found OSA in 22% of city bus and tram drivers, while in a similar population in western Iran 25% had a moderate to severe form of the disease. In Malaysia [107], 29% of bus drivers were confirmed to have mild, 9% moderate, and 7% severe OSA, which is significantly higher than the OSA risk estimated by the BQ in the same study (14.6%).

Firat et al. [118] in a sample of 90 drivers in Turkey found moderate and severe OSA in more than half of the subjects, and age and obesity played a significant role. In a study performed on 100 commercial drivers in Serbia [111], our study group confirmed OSA in 57% of subjects, with 11% having moderate, and 12% severe OSA (AHI > 30/h).

One of the largest studies of OSA in commercial drivers included nearly 20.000 subjects employed by companies that implemented mandatory OSA screening, diagnosis, and treatment programs [119]. An online screening tool identified 30% as having high risk for OSA, while subsequent PSG led to the diagnosis of OSA in 80% of those high-risk drivers.

These data on the prevalence of OSA in commercial drivers seem extremely worrying, especially when compared to the prevalence estimates of OSA in the general working-age (adult) population. It must be taken into account that the population of commercial drivers is under more frequent and detailed medical supervision compared to the general population, so the risk of having an unrecognized form of OSA should be significantly lower than in the general working population.

4.1 OSA and traffic accidents of commercial drivers

The frequency of excessive daytime sleepiness and OSA is significantly higher in the population of commercial drivers, especially bus and truck drivers, where the prevalence of moderate to severe OSA reaches 26–70% depending on the study [90, 120, 121].

There are several explanations such as a) the dominance of men in the profession, b) the high prevalence of OSA risk factors (middle and older age, obesity, alcohol and cigarette consumption, and accompanying diseases), c) additional risk factors (long working hours, shift work, and inadequate conditions for rest between shifts).

The first studies on the presence of OSA and the occurrence of traffic accidents in the population of commercial drivers appeared in the early 1990s. Stoohs et al. [112] found that 46% of truck drivers had sleep-disordered breathing. Drivers with OSA had more accidents compared to other drivers, but the difference was not statistically significant.

Howard et al. [113] surveyed more than 2000 commercial drivers in Australia and performed PSG on a subsample of 161 drivers. They found 24% of sleepy drivers in the sample and subsample, 60% of drivers had OSA (AHI > 5) and 16% of drivers had symptomatic OSA (AHI > 5, ESS > 11). The main risk factors for the accidents were excessive drowsiness and the use of drugs with a sedative effect.

In 2004, Alan Pack et al. published the results of a study on the influence of sleep length and OSA on the sleepiness and performance of commercial drivers [115]. The prevalence of OSA was about 28%, but the main risk factor for sleepiness was the length of sleep, not the severity of OSA. In a 2012 study [116], Sharwood et al. analyzed long-haul truck drivers in Australia and found that a small number of drivers (12%) reported excessive daytime sleepiness, and that OSA was present in 43% of respondents. In addition, 4.4% reported previously diagnosed OSA, but only half of them used the prescribed therapy.

Karimi et al. found OSA in 22% of respondents in a sample of public transport drivers in Gothenburg [117], and the frequency of traffic accidents was higher in this subgroup compared to the control. In newly diagnosed cases of OSA, therapeutic measures (CPAP or oral appliance) were applied, which showed a positive effect on the reduction of sleepiness and improvement of the subjects' neurocognitive abilities.

In a systematic review and meta study of the presence of drowsiness and the risk of traffic accidents in the population of commercial drivers [122], Zhang et al. analyzed the influence of acute drowsiness, presence of OSA and insomnia. They found that all investigated variables except insomnia had a moderate influence on the occurrence of traffic accidents, with the odds-ratio in the range of 1.72–1.85, which is significantly lower compared to non-commercial drivers. Luzzi et al. reported more than double risk of car accidents in commercial drivers with OSA compared to controls, but no significant correlation was found between sleepiness and car crashes [123].

4.2 OSA and work ability assessment of commercial drivers

The large number of studies indicating a link between OSA and traffic accidents raised the question whether it is necessary to perform OSA screening in high-risk occupational groups such as commercial drivers [124].

One of the most important questions is how to determine which drivers are at the highest risk of obstructive sleep apnea. The main reasons are, on the one hand, the limited availability and cost of the diagnostic procedure (PSG), and on the other hand, the legal obligation to recognize and treat OSA in commercial drivers in order to maintain their employment and reduce trauma. Therefore, there is great interest from employers and legislators, as well as from drivers themselves, in finding a quality modality for OSA screening or diagnosis. That ideal diagnostic modality should have high sensitivity and high specificity, be easy to apply, and not take too much work time and money.

Existing models for the prediction of OSA in commercial drivers are often based on the application of questionnaires for self-assessment of risk, such as the ESS, BQ, the STOP-BANG diagnostic model, and others [110, 118, 125–128]. Another type of model is based on the consensus criteria of groups of experts, which were later tested in practice [129–132]. The third approach is forming a model based on the clinical research results, as is the was the case in our study [113, 115, 116, 118, 119, 133, 134]. There are also the so-called complex statistical models based on clinical data, which have not yet been adequately tested in commercial drivers [135, 136].

The problem of the usability of the ESS scale as a screening OSA tool among commercial drivers has been recognized in previous research. There is a difference in data obtained through anonymous surveys, and data during driver's work ability testing. In the study by Parks et al. [129], which included 456 commercial vehicle drivers who came for a driver's license examination, the average ESS score was extremely low, 3.2 ± 2.7, and in a similar study by Talmage and associates [130] in a sample of nearly 1500 drivers, the ESS score ranged from 2.68–5.57, with only one driver reporting an ESS ≥ 10. In a large anonymous survey conducted in 2012 across all US transportation sectors [101], the average ESS score of truck and bus drivers was 5.2–5.7 (±4.4), with 10–15% reporting excessive sleepiness. A recent study in Japan, which analyzed data from almost 20.000 commercial drivers, using ESS as a screening tool and type IV device as a diagnostic tool, showed that sleepiness was associated with OSA severity, with low sensitivity and high specificity, with an improvement in sensitivity when adding BMI ≥ 25 kg/m^2 [137].

In 2004, Gurubhagavatula et al. [138]. proposed a two-stage model for detecting commercial drivers at high risk of OSA. In the first step, the model included the presence of symptoms and a high BMI, and in the second step, all-night oximetry. The model had a sensitivity and specificity of 91% for determining severe OSA. This study also pointed out that excessive sleepiness was not a mandatory element of OSA diagnosis, given the fact that drivers ability to maintain employment often depended on these data.

Huhta et al. [139] explored the BAMSA score (BMI > 30 kg m^{-2}, age > 50 years, male gender, snoring at least one night per week, and the presence of apnea at least sometimes) in more than 2000 drivers in Finland and found a sensitivity of 85.7% and a specificity of 78.8% in detecting AHI ≥ 15 when using a cut-off point of 4.

Tzischinsky et al. [140] used a set of questionnaires and the WatchPat-100 to confirm OSA in candidates for a professional driver's license. Using logistic regression, they found that BMI, age, smoking, information about snoring in the family, and falling asleep while driving but as a passenger, the best predictors of OSA.

In a study performed on 100 commercial drivers in Serbia, with the use of standardized questionnaires, compared to the results of PSG or HSAT, our study group found that the main indicators of OSA (AHI ≥ 5/h) were STOP-BANG score greater than 5, presence of lung disease, abdominal obesity and night work, while the more severe form of the disease (AHI ≥ 15/h), in addition to STOP-BANG≥5 and abdominal obesity, was also indicated by presence of self reported excessive sleepiness (ESS ≥ 10), prolonged work, medication use, and the diagnosis of periodic limb movements during sleep. Each of the above factors approximately doubled the odds of having OSA [141].

During 2006, a joint recommendation [142] of several professional and non-governmental associations of medical specialists (American College of Chest Physicians, American College of Occupational and Environmental Medicine, National Sleep Foundation) was published on the elements for initial and periodic examinations of commercial drivers in case of suspected OSA, and work ability assessment of drivers with confirmed OSA. The main assessment parameters were excessive daytime sleepiness, clinical signs of OSA, high BMI, neck circumference and arterial hypertension, with suggested PSG for OSA confirmation. Until the diagnosis of OSA was confirmed, the driver was unable to work. If OSA is confirmed, continuous application of adequate therapy (CPAP, oral appliances, surgical intervention) was necessary to restore the driver's commercial vehicle license.

In 2016, the US Federal Motor Carrier Safety Administration and the Federal Railroad Administration proposed mandatory guidelines addressing OSA in commercial drivers and rail operators based on earlier recommendations and guidelines from 2012 [143]. The criteria for referring drivers to PSG were BMI > 35 kg/m2, symptoms and signs (snoring, interruptions in breathing during sleep, and excessive sleepiness), and other OSA risk factors (small or retracted jaw, reduced pharyngeal space, hypertension, diabetes, hypothyroidism, etc.). The cut-off for mandatory therapy was AHI > 20, and the therapy of choice was CPAP for at least 4 hours every night for 70% of the nights. These guidelines met with great criticism, primarily because of the significant PSG costs, which in most cases had to be covered by the drivers themselves. Unfortunately, the proposal was declined in 2017 [144].

In 2020, Burks et al. [145] analyzed the usefulness of commercial driver medical examination (CDME) screening criteria for OSA in comparison to PSG findings and found that CDME identified only 20.7% of the drivers later diagnosed with moderate or severe OSA, with 86% specificity, modest positive predictive value, and low negative predictive value was low. An interesting finding was seen in the subset of drivers that were diagnosed with moderate to severe OSA before CDME, treated with CPAP and instructed to report the condition on CDME. Almost 30% of the commercial drivers with OSA decided not to report the condition when asked and received a longer certification license than subjects who disclosed their CPAP use.

In 2022, the American academy of sleep medicine (AASM) has published their position statement on screening, diagnosing, and treating OSA in the transportation sector [146]. They have recognized that OSA occurs at a high prevalence in commercial drivers and other transportation operators, and that the adequate screening, diagnosis, and treatment leads to prevention of OSA-related traffic accidents, comorbidities and economic costs. The screening procedure should take into account the objective parameters (hypertension and BMI) even in absence of subjective parameters (excessive sleepiness), while work ability (fitness to drive) must be determined with adequate diagnosis and treatment and through discussion with the patient, their family members, and eventually state driver licensing agency representatives.

Several large transportation companies understood the importance of adequate OSA screening diagnosis and treatment of commercial drivers and the impact on traffic accidents and costs of work and life and implemented OSA programs [119]. A recently published report analyzed the safety benefits of two, carrier-implemented OSA programs for commercial drivers and found a dose response benefit according to CPAP use in OSA drivers and the largest benefit in fully compliant commercial drivers who had an accident prior to OSA diagnosis [147].

In the countries of the European Union, from 01.07.2014, a Directive 2014/85/EU was implemented, placing OSA on the list of diseases of importance for driving a motor vehicle [148]. According to this directive, a driver candidate with suspected moderate (AHI 15–30/h) or severe OSA (AHI > 30/h) must be referred for examination by a specialist doctor, that is, for possible confirmation of the diagnosis.

Patients diagnosed with moderate or severe OSA must regularly use the prescribed therapy and be checked at least once a year (commercial drivers) or once every 3 years (amateur drivers) if they want to keep their driving license.

The details of the OSA risk assessment methodology were later specified in a form of European Obstructive Sleep Apnea Screening (EUROSAS) questionnaire for drivers, which includes 11 items, four items on demographic characteristics (gender, age, weight, and height), six items refer to history of sleepiness while driving, having a serious accident due to sleepiness, history of snoring, witnessed apneas and non-restorative sleep, and high blood pressure. The final item is the ESS score. The value for the EUROSAS ranges from 2 to 24, with individuals with 10 points or above are considered OSA high risk and should be referred to a sleep specialist. The choice of confirmatory sleep diagnostic procedure or treatment are left to sleep specialists and patients to discuss [149].

There is a challenge of conducting the proper diagnostic procedure in commercial drivers due to legal and job loss related issues. The most comfortable and cost effective methods, such as HSAT cannot be used without some form of long distance video monitoring, since there is a possibility that the high risk driver would not perform the study properly (inadequate/insufficient result), or would put the diagnostic device on other low –risk subject such as family member or a friend, leading to false-negative results and easier driving recertification procedure [145]. The newer procedures, with the possibility of several night recordings with smart devices, could be, with some modifications (personalized codes, recording in a controlled environment, etc.) the diagnostic procedure of choice for uncomplicated cases [49, 50].

5. OSA and other high risk occupations

A systematic review and meta- analysis on occupation and OSA has revealed a well-known correlation between OSA and commercial drivers and also a significant OSA risk in organic solvents occupational exposure industries [150].

A meta-analysis published in 2022 dealt with the prevalence of sleep disorders, including OSA, in the first responders' professions, and found a pooled OSA prevalence of 30% among first responders for medical emergencies, which correlated with the presence of cardiovascular, metabolic, and psychiatric disorders [151].

In a recent prospective study from Izmir [152], almost 1000 male middle-aged heavy machinery operators were screened for OSA by using STOP BANG questionnaire, with 142 identified as high risk for OSA. PSG study was performed in 110 of those subjects and revealed a presence of OSA in more than 60%, with 32% mild, 18% moderate, and 13% severe OSA. The presence of OSA was compared with employer registered accidents at work, showing a statistically significant relationship between the accident rate and OSA severity.

In a cross-sectional study of 328 commercial airline pilots from three commercial companies, OSA risk by Berlin Questionnaire was high in 30%, excessive daytime sleepiness (ESS > 10) was reported by 34% of pilots, while 45% had fallen asleep while in control of the plane [153]. In a study on OSA prevalence in Saudi commercial pilots and first officers [154], 69% had OSA, with 5% having moderate to severe OSA determined by HSAT. 23% were excessively sleepy during the day.

There were several cases of railroad traffic accidents with heavy casualties caused by railroad operators falling asleep, but mandatory OSA screening of railway personnel is in many countries rare or triggered by the accident [155]. The study performed on more than 700 male railroad workers in Brazil showed high risk of OSA by BQ and confirmed OSA in 35% of subjects [156]. Australian National Standard for Health Assessment of Rail Safety Workers introduced screening for OSA in safety critical rail workers in 2004 by using the ESS score as the main parameter. The estimated prevalence of OSA by using self-reported sleepiness was only 2%, suggesting under-diagnosis of OSA. The Australian standard was updated in 2012 and besides ESS, included objective parameters such as high BMI, type 2 diabetes, hypertension requiring two or more medications, history of habitual loud snoring or witnessed apnea in sleep. A study based on the new criteria has analyzed more than 4000 subjects, revealing a joint OSA prevalence (previously or newly diagnosed) of 7% in railroad workers. Out of 200 high risk workers, sleep studies have confirmed OSA in 91% [157].

A study performed in active US military personnel [158], recognized 393,857 new cases of OSA from 2005 to 2016, with the significant raise in the OSA incidence rates (per 10,000 subjects) going from 11.8 in 2005 to 333.8 in 2016. The average service member with newly diagnosed OSA was middle-aged male, white, married, and working in the Army sector. OSA often appears together with insomnia (Comorbid OSA and insomnia, COMISA) in active duty military personnel [159]. The prevalence in active army pilots is around 3%, which appears lower than in general population, but is still very high taking into consideration the level and frequency of medical fitness to work assessment protocols in these specific high-risk population [160].

In the current guidelines for screening and diagnosing OSA and insomnia in military personnel, the authors recommended STOP questionnaire, followed by manually scored HSAT. For patients who have non-diagnostic HSAT, repeated testing (HSAT or PSG) should be done [161].

6. Conclusion

Sleep disorders are very prevalent in the adult working population especially in the current concept of 24/7 modern society and if left unrecognized or untreated can lead to serious consequences on health and quality of sleep and life.

Sleep-related breathing disorders, especially OSA, have slowly but steadily become one of the leading chronic non-communicable diseases, affecting almost one billion people worldwide, with at least 400 million people in need of urgent treatment. Unfortunately, due to inadequate education of the healthcare workers and general population, and limited diagnostic facilities, it is estimated that more than 80% patients are still unaware of their illness or untreated.

The current scientific knowledge recognizes the strong association of OSA and excessive daytime sleepiness, accidents and injuries at work, traffic accidents, as well as cardiovascular, respiratory, metabolic, neurological, psychiatric, and malignant diseases.

The costs of human lives, diagnosing and treating injuries and comorbidities, other material and non-material costs caused by not recognizing and treating OSA are getting higher by the day reaching billions of dollars annually.

One of the most vulnerable populations are people working in high-risk occupations, such as transportation of people and goods (commercial truck and bus drivers, pilots, and railroad operators), heavy machinery operators, first responders (police, firemen, and paramedics), and military personnel.

Long and unpredictable working hours, shift work, night work, stress levels, exposure to physical, chemical and biological hazards often lead to inadequate nutrition, rest and reduced availability of healthcare of the employees. On the other hand, their job demands leave a very small space for mistakes, with a high chance of placing themselves or others at risk of injury in the event of poor performance.

The estimated prevalence of OSA in high risk occupations is significantly higher than in general population, as well as the consequences. Mandatory medical screening for disorders that can affect fitness to work in these occupations are part of legislation in many countries worldwide. Sleep disorders and OSA are usually mentioned as a part of broad category of illnesses that can affect work ability (for example, driving) with no specific questions or tests concerning sleep, sleepiness, and breathing during sleep. Most of the healthcare professionals lack standardized education on sleep-related breathing disorders and avoid discussing the issue with their patients or examinees. The specific challenge is the attitude of people working in high risk professions, who, driven by fear of losing their jobs or benefits, do not mention or decide not to report sleep-related issues (sleepiness or falling asleep while driving, operating machinery, and work at height) or previously diagnosed or even treated disorders.

The technological advances, followed by a strong demand (many patients, limited diagnostic capacities) have led to development of easy to use OSA diagnostic devices (high-end commercial wrist watches), which, in combination with telemedicine, significantly reduced the costs and time from suspicion to diagnosis and adequate treatment of OSA. CPAP devices, although still treatment of choice for many patients, are not the only treatment modality, making it possible for patients to find the best and most comfortable solution for their disease.

Today, many of the obstacles on the road to fast, not expensive and adequate diagnosis and treatment of sleep-related breathing disorders have been eliminated.

There is still a great need for raising awareness in employees, employers, healthcare providers, and communities through education on the significance, proper diagnostic and treatment solutions, as well as consequences of untreated OSA in the high-risk occupations and safety sensitive jobs. There is a strong demand for updating or creating new fitness to work assessment protocols and legislation covering health and safety and driving in order to implement proper preventive measures and reduce the burden of OSA and other sleep-related breathing disorders.

Conflict of interest

The author declares no conflict of interest.

Author details

Martin Popević[1,2]

1 Institute of Occupational Health Military Medical Academy, Belgrade, Serbia

2 Faculty of Medicine, University of Defense, Belgrade, Serbia

*Address all correspondence to: popevic.martin@gmail.com

References

[1] Carskadon MA, Dement WC. Normal human sleep: An overview. In: Kryger MH, Roth T, Dement WC, editors. Principles and Practice of Sleep Medicine. 6th ed. Philadelphia, PA: Elsevier Saunders; 2017. pp. 15-24

[2] Buysse DJ. Sleep health: Can we define it? Does it matter? Sleep. 2014;**37**(1):9-17

[3] Morin CM, Jarrin DC. Epidemiology of insomnia: Prevalence, course, risk factors, and public health burden. Sleep Medicine Clinics. 2022;**17**(2):173-191

[4] Bansil P, Kuklina EV, Merritt RK, Yoon PW. Associations between sleep disorders, sleep duration, quality of sleep, and hypertension: Results from the National Health and nutrition examination survey, 2005 to 2008. The Journal of Clinical Hypertension. 2011;**13**(10):739-743

[5] Jaqua EE, Hanna M, Labib W, Moore C, Matossian V. Common sleep disorders affecting older adults. The Permanente Journal. 2023;**27**(1):122

[6] Rowley JA, Safwan BM. Normal sleep. In: Safwan BM, editor. Essentials of Sleep Medicine. Respiratory Medicine. Switzerland AG: Springer Nature; 2022. DOI: 10.1007/978-3-030-93739-3_1

[7] Sahlman J. Obstructive sleep apnea in adults evolution, and related inflammation in early stages of disease [doctoral thesis]. Faculty of Health Sciences, University of Eastern Finland: Kuopio. 2011

[8] American Academy of Sleep Medicine: International Classification of Sleep Disorders: 3rd. Text revision. American Academy of Sleep Medicine, 2023

[9] Thorpy MJ, Billiard M, editors. Sleep disorders and excessive sleepiness. In: Sleepiness: Causes, Consequences and Treatment. Cambridge, UK: Cambridge University Press; 2011

[10] Javaheri S, Badr MS. Central sleep apnea: Pathophysiologic classification. Sleep. 2023;**46**(3):zsac 113

[11] Verbraecken J. Sleep related breathing disorders. In: Claudio B et al., editors. Nosological Classification, Definitions and Epidemiology. Regensburg, Germany: ESRS Sleep Medicine Textbook; 2021. pp. 297-310

[12] Epstein LJ, Kristo D, Strollo PJ Jr, Friedman N, Malhotra A, Patil SP, et al Adult obstructive sleep apnea task force of the American Academy of sleep medicine. Clinical guideline for the evaluation, management and long-term care of obstructive sleep apnea in adults. Journal of Clinical Sleep Medicine. 2009;**5**(3):263-276

[13] Rapoport DM. Point: Is the AHI the best way to quantify the severity of sleep disordered breathing?-Yes. Chest. Jan 2016;**149**(1):14-16. DOI: 10.1378/chest.15-1319

[14] Punjabi NM. Counterpoint: Is the ahi the best way to quantify the severity of sleep disordered breathing? No. Chest. Jan 2016;**149**(1):16-19. DOI: 10.1378/chest.14-2261

[15] Rapoport DM. Rebuttal from Dr. Rapoport. Chest. Jan 2016;**149**(1):19-20. DOI: 10.1378/chest.15-1320

[16] Malhotra A, Ayappa I, Ayas N, Collop N, Kirsch D, Mcardle N, et al. Metrics of sleep apnea severity: Beyond the apnea-hypopnea index. Sleep. 2021;**44**(7):zsab030

[17] Kendzerska T, Mollayeva T, Gershon AS, Leung RS, Hawker G, Tomlinson G. Untreated obstructive sleep apnea and the risk for serious long-term adverse outcomes: A systematic review. Sleep Medicine Reviews. 2014;**18**(1):49-59

[18] Peppard PE, Young T, Barnett JH, Palta M, Hagen EW, Hla KM. Increased prevalence of sleep-disordered breathing in adults. American Journal of Epidemiology. 2013;**177**:1006-1014

[19] Heinzer R, Watt S, Marques-Vidal P, Marti-Soler H, Andries D, Tobback N, et al. Prevalence of sleep-disordered breathing in the general population: The HypnoLaus study. The Lancet Respiratory Medicine. 2015;**3**(4):310-318

[20] Benjafield AV, Ayas NT, Eastwood PR, Heinzer R, Ip MSM, Morrell MJ, et al. Estimation of the global prevalence and burden of obstructive sleep apnoea: A literature-based analysis. The Lancet Respiratory Medicine. 2019;**7**:687-698

[21] Tishler PV, Larkin EK, Schluchter MD, Redline S. Incidence of sleep-disordered breathing in an urban adult population: The relative importance of risk factors in the development of sleep-disordered breathing. The Payment. 2003;**289**(17):2230-2237

[22] Lyons MM, Bhatt NY, Pack AI, Magalang UJ. Global burden of sleep-disordered breathing and its implications. Respirology. 2020;**25**(7):690-702. DOI: 10.1111/resp.13838. Epub 2020 May 21

[23] Rowley JA, Safwan BM. Anatomy and physiology of upper airway obstruction. In: Kryger MH, Roth T, Dement WC, editors. Principles and Practice of Sleep Medicine. 6th ed. Philadelphia, PA: Elsevier Saunders; 2017. pp. 1076-1087

[24] Zhao Y, Tao L, Nie P, Lu X, Xu X, Chen J, et al. Association between 5-HT2A receptor polymorphisms and risk of obstructive sleep apnea and hypopnea syndrome: A systematic review and meta-analysis. Gene. 2013;**530**(2):287-294

[25] Jordan AS, McSharry DG, Malhotra A. Adult obstructive sleep apnea. The Lancet. 2014;**383**(9918): 736-747

[26] Veatch OJ, Bauer CR, Keenan BT, et al. Characterization of genetic and phenotypic heterogeneity of obstructive sleep apnea using electronic health records. BMC Medical Genomics. 2020;**13**:105. DOI: 10.1186/s12920-020-00755-4

[27] Caporale M, Palmeri R, Corallo F, et al. Cognitive impairment in obstructive sleep apnea syndrome: A descriptive review. Sleep & Breathing. 2021;**25**:29-40. DOI: 10.1007/s11325-020-02084-3

[28] Abrishami A, Khajehdehi A, Chung F. A systematic review of screening questionnaires for obstructive sleep apnea. Canadian Journal of Anesthesia/Journal Canadien d'anesthesie. 2010;**57**(5):423-438

[29] Zhang C, Berger MB, Rielly A, Malhotra A, Kales SN. Obstructive sleep apnea in the workplace. In: Principles and Practice of Sleep Medicine. Philadelphia, USA: Elsevier; 2017. pp. 750-756

[30] Netzer NC, Stoohs RA, Netzer CM, Clark K, Strohl KP. Using the Berlin questionnaire to identify patients at risk for the sleep apnea syndrome. Annals of Internal Medicine. 1999;**131**:485-491

[31] Bouloukaki et al. Translation and validation of the Berlin questionnaire

in primary health care in Greece. BMC Pulmonary Medicine. 2013;**13**:6

[32] Sharma SK, Vasudev C, Sinha S, Banga A, Pandey RM, Hande K. Validation of the modified Berlin questionnaire to identify patients at risk for the obstructive sleep apnea syndrome. Indian Journal of Medical Research. 2006;**124**(3):281-290

[33] Chung F, Yegneswaran B, Liao P, Chung SA, Vairavanathan S, Islam S, et al. Validation of the Berlin questionnaire and American Society of Anesthesiologists checklist as screening tools for obstructive sleep apnea in surgical patients. The Journal of the American Society of Anesthesiologists. 2008;**108**(5):822-830

[34] Gus M, Gonçalves SC, Martinez D, de Abreu Silva EO, Moreira LB, Fuchs SC, et al. Risk for obstructive sleep apnea by Berlin questionnaire, but not daytime sleepiness, is associated with resistant hypertension: A case–control study. American Journal of Hypertension. 2008;**21**(7):832-835

[35] Chilukuri K, Dalal D, Marine JE, Scherr D, Henrikson CA, Cheng A, et al. Predictive value of obstructive sleep apnea assessed by the Berlin questionnaire for outcomes after the catheter ablation of atrial fibrillation. Europace. 2009;**11**(7):896-901

[36] Ahmadi N, Chung SA, Gibbs A, Shapiro CM. The Berlin questionnaire for sleep apnea in a sleep clinic population: Relationship to polysomnographic measurement of respiratory disturbance. Sleep & Breathing. 2008;**12**(1):39-45

[37] Vaz AP, Drummond M, Mota PC, Severo M, Almeida J, Winck JC. Translation of Berlin questionnaire to Portuguese language and its application in OSA identification in a sleep disordered breathing clinic. Revista Portuguesa de Pneumologia. 2011;**17**:59-65

[38] Chung F, Yegneswaran B, Liao P, Chung SA, Vairavanathan S, Islam S, et al. STOP questionnaire: A tool to screen patients for obstructive sleep apnea. Anesthesiology. 2008;**108**:812-821

[39] Chung F, Subramanyam R, Liao P, Sasaki E, Shapiro C, Sun Y. High STOP-Bang score indicates a high probability of obstructive sleep apnea. British Journal of Anaesthesia. 2012;**108**(5):768-775. DOI: 10.1093/bja/aes022

[40] Silva GE, Vana KD, Goodwin JL, Sherrill DL, Quan SF. Identification of patients with sleep disordered breathing: Comparing the four-variable screening tool, STOP, STOP-BANG, and Epworth sleepiness scales. Journal of Clinical Sleep Medicine. 2011;7(5):467-472

[41] Dias RA, Hardin KA, Rose H, Agius MA, Apperson ML, Brass SD. Sleepiness, fatigue, and risk of obstructive sleep apnea using the STOP-BANG questionnaire in multiple sclerosis: A pilot study. Sleep & Breathing. 2012;**16**:1255-1265

[42] Nicholl DDM, Ahmed SB, Loewen AHS, Hemmelgarn BR, Sola DY, Beecroft JM, et al. Diagnostic value of screening instruments for identifying obstructive sleep apnea in kidney failure. Journal of Clinical Sleep Medicine. 2013;**9**(1):31-38

[43] Boynton G, Vahabzadeh A, Hammoud S, Ruzicka DL, Chervin RD. Validation of the STOP-BANG questionnaire among patients referred for suspected obstructive sleep apnea. Journal of Sleep Disorders–Treatment and Care. 2013;**2**(4):23. DOI: 10.4172/2325-9639.1000121

[44] Gibson GJ. Obstructive sleep apnea syndrome: Underestimated and undertreated. British Medical Bulletin. 2005;**72**:49-64

[45] Geyer JD, Talathi S, Carney PR. Introduction to sleep and polysomnography. In: John L, Greenfield JR, Geyer JD, Carney PR, editors. Reading EEGs: A Practical Approach. Philadelphia: Lippincott Williams & Wilkins; 2009

[46] Kushida CA, Littner MR, Morgenthaler T, Alessi CA, Bailey D, Coleman J Jr, et al. Practice parameters for the indications for polysomnography and related procedures: An update for 2005. Sleep. 2005;**28**(4):499-521

[47] Pinna GD, Robbi E, Pizza F, Taurino AE, Pronzato C, La Rovere MT, et al. Can cardiorespiratory polygraphy replace portable polysomnography in the assessment of sleep-disordered breathing in heart failure patients? Sleep and Breathing. 2014;**18**(3):475-482

[48] Caples SM, Anderson WM, Calero K, Howell M, Hashmi SD. Use of polysomnography and home sleep apnea tests for the longitudinal management of obstructive sleep apnea in adults: An American Academy of sleep medicine clinical guidance statement. Journal of Clinical Sleep Medicine. 2021;**17**(6):1287-1293

[49] Pépin JL, Letesson C, Le-Dong NN, Dedave A, Denison S, Cuthbert V, et al. Assessment of mandibular movement monitoring with machine learning analysis for the diagnosis of obstructive sleep apnea. JAMA Network Open. 2020;**3**(1):e1919657

[50] Browne SH, Vaida F, Umlauf A, Kim J, DeYoung P, Owens RL. Performance of a commercial smart watch compared to polysomnography reference for overnight continuous oximetry measurement and sleep apnea evaluation. Journal of Clinical Sleep Medicine. 2024;**20**(9):1479-1488. DOI: 10.5664/jcsm.11178

[51] Kapur VK, Auckley DH, Chowdhuri S, Kuhlmann DC, Mehra R, Ramar K, et al. Clinical practice guideline for diagnostic testing for adult obstructive sleep apnea: An American Academy of sleep medicine clinical practice guideline. Journal of Clinical Sleep Medicine. 2017;**13**(3):479-504

[52] Pataka A, Daskalopoulou E, Kalamaras G, Passa KF, Argyropoulou P. Evaluation of five different questionnaires for assessing sleep apnea syndrome in a sleep clinic. Sleep Medicine. 2014;**15**(7):776-781

[53] El-Sayed IH. Comparison of four sleep questionnaires for screening obstructive sleep apnea. Egyptian Journal of Chest Diseases and Tuberculosis. 2012;**61**(4):433-441

[54] Freedman N. Positive airway pressure treatment for obstructive sleep Apnea. In: Kryger MH, Roth T, Dement WC, editors. Principles and Practice of Sleep Medicine. 6th ed. Philadelphia, PA: Elsevier Saunders; 2017. pp. 1125-1137

[55] Patil SP, Ayappa IA, Caples SM, Kimoff RJ, Patel SR, Harrod CG. Treatment of adult obstructive sleep apnea with positive airway pressure: An American Academy of sleep medicine clinical practice guideline. Journal of Clinical Sleep Medicine. 2019;**15**(2):335-343

[56] Ramar K, Dort LC, Katz SG, Lettieri CJ, Harrod CG, Thomas SM, et al. Clinical practice guideline for the treatment of obstructive sleep apnea

and snoring with oral appliance therapy: An update for 2015. Journal of Clinical Sleep Medicine. 2015;**11**(7):773-827

[57] Vukoje N. Cut for Peaceful Sleep - Let's Defeat Snoring. Sremski Karlovci: Novi Sad. Zoran Stojanović Publishing House; 2008

[58] Kent D, Stanley J, Aurora RN, et al. Referral of adults with obstructive sleep apnea for surgical consultation: An American Academy of sleep medicine clinical practice guideline. Journal of Clinical Sleep Medicine. 2021;**17**(12):2499-2505

[59] Schütz SG, Dunn A, Braley TJ, Pitt B, Shelgikar AV. New frontiers in pharmacologic obstructive sleep apnea treatment: A narrative review. Sleep Medicine Reviews. 2021;**57**:101473

[60] Costantino A, Rinaldi V, Moffa A, Luccarelli V, Bressi F, Cassano M, et al. Hypoglossal nerve stimulation long-term clinical outcomes: A systematic review and meta-analysis. Sleep and Breathing. 2020;**24**:399-411

[61] Harańczyk M, Konieczyńska M, Płazak W. Endothelial dysfunction in obstructive sleep apnea patients. Sleep & Breathing. 2022;**26**:231-242. DOI: 10.1007/s11325-021-02382-4

[62] Kim S, Lee KY, Kim NH, Abbott RD, Kim C, Lee SK, et al. Relationship of obstructive sleep apnoea severity and subclinical systemic atherosclerosis. European Respiratory Journal. 2020;**55**(2).1900959. DOI: 10.1183/13993003.00959-2019

[63] Mitra AK, Bhuiyan AR, Jones EA. Association and risk factors for obstructive sleep apnea and cardiovascular diseases: A systematic review. Diseases. 2021;**9**(4):88. DOI: 10.3390/diseases9040088

[64] Brown J, Yazdi F, Jodari-Karimi M, Owen JG, Reisin E. Obstructive sleep apnea and hypertension: Updates to a critical relationship. Current Hypertension Reports. 2022;**24**(6):173-184

[65] Cozowicz C, Memtsoudis SG. Perioperative Management of the Patient with Obstructive Sleep Apnea: A narrative review. Anesthesia & Analgesia. 2021;**132**(5):1231-1243. DOI: 10.1213/ANE.0000000000005444

[66] Kapur VK, Baldwin CM, Resnick HE, et al. Sleepiness in patients with moderate to severe sleep-disordered breathing. Sleep. 2005;**28**:472-477

[67] Roure N, Gomez S, Mediano O, et al. Daytime sleepiness and polysomnography in obstructive sleep apnea patients. Sleep Medicine. 2008;**9**:727-731

[68] Sauter C, Assenbaum S, Popovic R, et al. Excessive daytime sleepiness in patients suffering from different levels of obstructive sleep apnea syndrome. Journal of Sleep Research. 2000;**9**:293-301

[69] Basta M, Lin HM, Pejovic S, Sarrigiannidis A, et al. Lack of regular exercise, depression, and degree of apnea are predictors of excessive daytime sleepiness in patients with sleep apnea: Sex differences. Journal of Clinical Sleep Medicine. 2008;**4**:19-25

[70] Gottlieb DJ, Yao Q, Redline S, Ali T, et al. Does snoring predict sleepiness independently of apnea and hypopnea frequency? American Journal of Respiratory and Critical Care Medicine. 2000;**162**:1512-1517

[71] Mediano O, Barcello A, de la Pena M, et al. Daytime sleepiness and polysomnographic variables in

sleep apnea patients. The European Respiratory Journal. 2007;**30**:110-113

[72] Vgontzas AN, Bixler EO, Chrousos G. Obesity-related sleepiness and fatigue: The role of the stress system and cytokines. Annals of the New York Academy of Sciences. 2006;**1083**:329-344

[73] Koutsourelakis I, Perraki E, Bonakis A. Determinants of subjective sleepiness in suspected obstructive sleep apnea. Journal of Sleep Research. 2008;**17**:437-443

[74] Ryan S, McNicholas WT. Intermittent hypoxia and activation of inflammatory molecular pathways in OSAS. Archives of Physiology and Biochemistry. 2008;**114**:261-266

[75] Arzt M, Young T, Peppard P, et al. Dissociation of obstructive sleep apnea from hypersomnolence and obesity in patients with stroke. Stroke. 2010;**41**:e129-e134

[76] Capodanno D, Cumbo M, Marchese A, et al. Daytime sleepiness does not predict sleep apnea in patients with coronary artery disease. International Journal of Cardiology. 2011;**151**:248-250

[77] Morrell MJ, Finn L, McMillan A, Peppard PE. The impact of aging and sex on the association between sleepiness and sleep disordered breathing. The European Respiratory Journal. 2012;**40**:386-393

[78] McDaid C, Durée KH, Griffin SC, et al. A systematic review of continuous positive airway pressure for obstructive sleep apnea–hypopnoea syndrome. Sleep Medicine Reviews. 2009;**13**:427-436

[79] Weaver T, Mancini C, Maislin G, et al. CPAP treatment of sleepy patients with milder OSA: Results of the CATNAP randomized clinical trial. American Journal of Respiratory and Critical Care Medicine. 2012;**186**:677-683

[80] Pépin JL, Viot-Blanc V, Escourrou P, et al. Prevalence of residual excessive sleepiness in CPAP-treated sleep apnea patients: The French multicentre study. The European Respiratory Journal. 2009;**33**:1062-1067

[81] Koutsourelakis I, Perraki E, Economou NT, et al. Predictors of residual sleepiness in adequately treated obstructive sleep apnea patients. The European Respiratory Journal. 2009;**34**:687-693

[82] Bucks R, Olaithe M, Eastwood P. Neurocognitive function in obstructive sleep apnea: A meta - Review. Respirology. 2013;**18**(1):61-70

[83] Gagnon K, Baril AA, Gagnon JF, Fortin M, Decary A, Lafond C, et al. Cognitive impairment in obstructive sleep apnea. Pathologie Biologie. 2014;**62**(5):233-240

[84] Guglielmi O, Jurado-Gámez B, Gude F, Buela-Casal G. Occupational health of patients with obstructive sleep apnea syndrome: A systematic review. Sleep and Breathing. Mar 2015;**19**:35-44. DOI: 10.1007/s11325-014-1015-8

[85] Uehli K, Mehta A, Miedinger D, Hug K, Schindler C, Holsboer-Trachsler E, et al. Sleep problems and work injuries: A systematic review and meta-analysis. Sleep Medicine Reviews. 2014;**18**(1):61-73

[86] Guilleminault C, Billiard M, Montplaisir J, Dement WC. Altered states of consciousness in disorders of daytime sleepiness. Journal of the Neurological Sciences. 1975;**26**(3):377-393

[87] Young T, Blustein J, Finn L. Sleep-disordered breathing and motor vehicle accidents in a population-based sample of employed adults. Sleep. 1997;**20**:608-601

[88] Ellen RL, Marshall SC, Palayew M, Molnar FJ, Wilson KG. Systematic review of motor vehicle crash risk in persons with sleep apnea. Journal of Clinical Sleep Medicine. 2006;**2**:193-200

[89] Sassani A, Findley L, Kryger M, Goldlust E, George C, Davidson T. Reducing motor vehicle collisions, costs, and fatalities by treating obstructive sleep apnea syndrome. Sleep. 2004;**27**:453-458

[90] Tregear S, Reston J, Schoelles K, Phillips B. Obstructive sleep apnea and risk of motor vehicle crash: Systematic review and meta analysis. Journal of Clinical Sleep Medicine. 2009;**5**(6):573-581

[91] Tregear S, Reston J, Schoelles K, Phillips B. Continuous positive airway pressure reduces risk of motor vehicle crash among drivers with obstructive sleep apnea; Systematic review and meta-analysis. Sleep. 2010;**33**:1373-1380

[92] Luzzi V, Mazur M, Guaragna M, Di Carlo G, Cotticelli L, Magliulo G, et al. Correlations of obstructive sleep apnea syndrome and daytime sleepiness with the risk of car accidents in adult working population: A systematic review and meta-analysis with a gender-based approach. Journal of Clinical Medicine. 2022;**11**(14):3971

[93] National Claims Compensation Helpline. Understanding High Risk Jobs: Exploring Professions and Environments. Posted on 16/09/2023. Available from: https://national-claims.co.uk/understanding-high-risk-jobs-exploring-professions-and-environments/

[94] Martin S. Determing fitness to work at safety sensitive jobs. BCMJ. 2010;**52**:48

[95] Directive 2003/59/EC of the European Parliament and of the council of 15 July 2003 on the initial qualification and periodic training of drivers of certain road vehicles for the carriage of goods or passengers, amending council regulation (EEC) No 3820/85 and council directive 31/439/EEC and repealing council directive 76/914/EEC. Official Journal of the European Union. EU Commission. 2003;**L226**:04-17

[96] United States Department of Transportation Federal Motor Carrier Safety Administration. Regulations: Commercial driver's license standards; requirements and penalties: Definitions. Available from: http://www.fmcsa.dot.gov/regulations/title49/section/383.5

[97] van der Beek AJ. World at work: Truck drivers. Occupational and Environmental Medicine. 2012;**69**(4):291-295

[98] International Labor Organization (ILO). International hazard datasheets on occupation. Driver, sales route (food products). Available from: http://www.ilo.org/wcmsp5/groups/public/---ed_protect/---protrav/---safework/documents/publication/wcms_186151.pdf

[99] International Labor Organization (ILO). International Hazard Datasheets on Occupation. Driver, Truck/Heavy. Available from: http://www.ilo.org/wcmsp5/groups/public/---ed_protect/---protrav/---safework/documents/publication/wcms_186282.pdf

[100] Belenky G, Hanowski R, Jovanis P. Fatigue and commercial motorcoach/bus driver safety. In: Expert Panel Report Presented to FMCSA. McLean, VA: Manila Consulting Group; 2013

[101] Johnson KD, Patel SR, Baur DM, Edens E, Sherry P, Malhotra A, et al. Association of sleep habits with accidents and near misses in United States transportation operators. Journal of Occupational and Environmental Medicine/American College of Occupational and Environmental Medicine. 2014;**56**(5):510-515

[102] Hanowski RJ, Hickman J, Fumero MC, Olson RL, Dingus TA. The sleep of commercial vehicle drivers under the 2003 hours-of-service regulations. Accident Analysis & Prevention. 2007;**39**(6):1140-1145

[103] European Transport Safety Council. The Role of Driver Fatigue in Commercial Road Transport Crashes. Brussels. European Transport Safety Council; 2001. Available from: http://etsc.eu/wp-content/uploads/therole-of-driver-fatigue-in-commercial-road-transport-crashes.pdf

[104] European Union regulation (EC) No. 561/2006 of the European Parliament and of the council of 15 March 2006 on the harmonization of certain social legislation relating to road transport and amending council regulations (EEC) No. 3821/85 and (EC) No. 2135/98 and repealing council regulation (EEC) No. 3820/85. Official Journal of the European Union. European Parliament, Council of the European Union; 2006. DOI: 10211.04.2006

[105] Moreno CR, Carvalho FA, Lorenzi C, Matuzaki LS, Prezotti S, Bighetti P, et al. High risk for obstructive sleep apnea in truck drivers estimated by the Berlin questionnaire: Prevalence and associated factors. Chronobiology International. 2004;**21**:871-879

[106] Amra B, Dorali R, Mortazavi S, Golshan M, Farajzadegan Z, Fietze I, et al. Sleep apnea symptoms and accident risk factors in Persian commercial vehicle drivers. Sleep & Breathing. 2012;**16**:187-191

[107] Wahida AB, Ilhamah O, Suffian AM, Aimi MF, Norlen M, Wong SV. Obstructive sleep apnea among commercial vehicle drivers in Malaysia: Issues and initiatives. Health. 2013;**5**(8):80-86

[108] Popević MB, Milovanović A, Nagorni-Obradović L, Nešić D, Milovanović J, Milovanović AP. Screening commercial drivers for obstructive sleep apnea: Translation and validation of Serbian version of Berlin questionnaire. Quality of Life Research. 2016;**25**(2):343-349. DOI: 10.1007/s11136-015-1087-3

[109] Chen L, Pivetta B, Nagappa M, Saripella A, Islam S, Englesakis M, et al. Validation of the STOP-Bang questionnaire for screening of obstructive sleep apnea in the general population and commercial drivers: A systematic review and meta-analysis. Sleep & Breathing. 2021;**25**(4):1741-1751. DOI: 10.1007/s11325-021-02299-y

[110] Ozder A, Gunay E, Eker HH, Ulasli SS. Excessive daytime sleepiness among Turkish public transportation drivers: A risk for road traffic accidents? Acta Medica. 2014;**30**:1121

[111] Popević MB, Milovanović A, Nagorni-Obradović L, Nešić D, Milovanović J, Milovanović AP. Screening commercial drivers for obstructive sleep apnea: Validation of STOP-BANG questionnaire. International Journal of Occupational Medicine and Environmental Health. 2017;**30**(5):751-761. DOI: 10.13075/ijomeh.1896.00906

[112] Stoohs RA, Guilleminault C, Itoi A, Dement WC. Traffic accidents in

commercial long-haul truck drivers: The influence of sleep-disordered breathing and obesity. Sleep. 1994;**17**:619-623

[113] Howard ME, Desai AV, Grunstein RR, Hukins C, Armstrong JG, Joffe D, et al. Sleepiness, sleep-disordered breathing, and accident risk factors in commercial vehicle drivers. American Journal of Respiratory and Critical Care Medicine. 2004;**170**:1014-1021

[114] Ting H, Huang RJ, Lai CH, Chang SW, Chung AH, Kuo TY, et al. Evaluation of candidate measures for home-based screening of sleep disordered breathing in Taiwanese bus drivers. Sensors. 2014;**14**:8126-8149

[115] Pack A, Maislin G, Staley B, et al. Impaired performance in commercial drivers: Role of sleep apnea and short sleep duration. American Journal Respiratory Critical Care Medicine. 2006;**174**:446-454

[116] Sharwood LN, Elkington J, Stevenson M, et al. Assessing sleepiness and sleep disorders in Australian long-distance commercial vehicle drivers: Self-report versus an "at home" monitoring device. Sleep. 2012;**35**:469-475

[117] Karimi M, Eder DN, Eskandari D, Zou D, Hedner JA, Grote L. Impaired vigilance and increased accident rate in public transport operators is associated with sleep disorders. Accident Analysis & Prevention. 2013;**51**:208-214

[118] Firat H, Yuceege M, Demir A, Ardic S. Comparison of four established questionnaires to identify highway bus drivers at risk for obstructive sleep apnea in Turkey. Sleep and Biological Rhythms. 2012;**10**(3):231-236

[119] Berger M, Varvarigou V, Rielly A, Czeisler CA, Malhotra A, Kales SN. Employer-mandated sleep apnea screening and diagnosis in commercial drivers. Journal of Occupational and Environmental Medicine. 2012;**54**(8):1017-1025

[120] Vennelle M, Engleman HM, Douglas NJ. Sleepiness and sleep-related accidents in commercial bus drivers. Sleep and Breathing. 2010;**14**(1):39-42

[121] Adami A, Tonon D, Corica A, et al. Poor performance of screening questionnaires for obstructive sleep apnea in male commercial drivers. Sleep & Breathing. 2022;**26**:541-547. DOI: 10.1007/s11325-021-02414-z

[122] Zhang T, Chan AHS. Sleepiness and the risk of road accidents for professional drivers: A systematic review and meta-analysis of retrospective studies. Safety Science. 2014;**70**:180-188

[123] Luzzi V, Mazur M, Guaragna M, Di Carlo G, Cotticelli L, Magliulo G, et al. Correlations of obstructive sleep apnea syndrome and daytime sleepiness with the risk of car accidents in adult working population: A systematic review and meta-analysis with a gender-based approach. Journal of Clinical Medicine. 2022;**11**:3971. DOI: 10.3390/jcm11143971

[124] Baumel M, Maislin G, Pack A. Population and occupational screening for obstructive sleep apnea: Are we there yet? American Journal of Respiratory and Critical Care Medicine. 1997;**155**(1):9-14

[125] Catarino R, Spratley J, Catarino I, Lunet N, Pais-Clemente M. Sleepiness and sleep-disordered breathing in truck drivers. Sleep and Breathing. 2014;**18**(1):59-68

[126] Ozoh OB, Okubadejo NU, Akanbi MO, Dania MG. High-risk of obstructive sleep apnea and excessive daytime sleepiness among commercial intra-city drivers in Lagos

metropolis. Nigerian Medical Journal. 2013;**54**(4):224-229

[127] Ramachandran SK, Josephs LA. A meta-analysis of clinical screening tests for obstructive sleep apnea. Anesthesiology. 2009;**110**(4):928-939

[128] Burns N. An integrative review of screening for obstructive sleep apnea in commercial vehicle drivers. Workplace Health & Safety. 2014;**62**(3):114-120

[129] Parks PD, Durand G, Tsismenakis AJ, Vela-Bueno A, Kales SN. Screening for obstructive sleep apnea during commercial driver medical examinations. Journal of Occupational and Environmental Medicine. 2009;**51**(3):275-282

[130] Talmage JB, Hudson TB, Hegmann KT, Thiese MS. Consensus criteria for screening commercial drivers for obstructive sleep apnea: Evidence of efficacy. Journal of Occupational and Environmental Medicine. 2008;**50**(3):324-329

[131] Ancoli-Israel S, Czeisler CA, George CF, Guilleminault C, Pack AI. Obstructive sleep apnea and commercial motor vehicle driver safety. In: Plymouth Meeting. PA, USA: ECRI Institute; 2008. Available from: https://www.fmcsa.dot.gov/sites/fmcsa.dot.gov/files/docs/Sleep-MEP-Panel-Recommendations-508.pdf

[132] Xie W, Chakrabarty S, Levine R, Johnson R, Talmage JB. Factors associated with obstructive sleep apnea among commercial motor vehicle drivers. Journal of Occupational and Environmental Medicine. 2011;**53**(2):169-173

[133] Maislin G, Pack AI, Kribbs NB, Smith PL, Schwartz AR, Kline LR, et al. A survey screen for prediction of apnea. Sleep. 1995;**18**(3):158-166

[134] Rowley JA, Aboussouan LS, Badr MS. The use of clinical prediction formulas in the evaluation of obstructive sleep apnea. Sleep-New York. 2000;**23**(7):929-942

[135] Eiseman NA, Westover MB, Mietus JE, Thomas RJ, Bianchi MT. Classification algorithms for predicting sleepiness and sleep apnea severity. Journal of Sleep Research. 2012;**21**(1):101-112

[136] Su CT, Chen KH, Chen LF, Wang PC, Hsiao YH. Prediagnosis of obstructive sleep apnea via multiclass MTS. Computational and Mathematical Methods in Medicine. 2012;**2012**(1):212498

[137] Wada H, Nakano H, Sakurai S, Tanigawa T. Self-reported sleep tendency poorly predicts the presence of obstructive sleep apnea in commercial truck drivers. Sleep Medicine. 2024;**115**:109-113

[138] Gurubhagavatula I, Maislin G, Nkwuo JE, Pack AI. Occupational screening for obstructive sleep apnea in commercial drivers. American Journal of Respiratory and Critical Care Medicine. 2004;**170**:371-376

[139] Huhta R, Sieminski M, Hirvonen K, Partinen E, Partinen M. A new screening tool (BAMSA) for sleep apnea in male professional truck drivers. Journal of Clinical Medicine. 2024;**13**(2):522. DOI: 10.3390/jcm13020522

[140] Tzischinsky O, Cohen A, Doveh E, Epstein R, Ribak J, Klein D, et al. Screening for sleep disordered breathing among applicants for a professional driver's license. Journal of Occupational and Environmental Medicine. 2012;**54**(10):1275-1280

[141] Popevic M. Sleepiness, obstructive sleep apnoea syndrome and traffic

accidents of commercial vehicle drivers [dissertations & theses]. University of Belgrade (Serbia) ProQuest. 2015. 30957191

[142] Hartenbaum N, Collop N, Rosen I, et al. Sleep apnea and commercial motor vehicle operators: Statement from the joint task force of the American College of Chest Physicians, the American College of Occupational and Environmental Medicine, and the National Sleep Foundation. Chest. 2006;**130**(3):637-639

[143] MCSAC and MRB Task 11-05—Final report on obstructive sleep apnea (OSA). 2012. Available from: http://www.mrb.fmcsa.dot.gov/documents/Meetings2012/Task11-05FinalCoverLetterandReport_2-21-12.docx

[144] Department of Transportation. Notice of withdrawal of proposed rulemaking on evaluation of safety sensitive personnel for moderate-to-severe obstructive sleep apnea (OSA). Federal Register. 2017:37038-37039. Available from: https://www.gpo.gov/fdsys/pkg/FR-2017-08-08/pdf/2017-16451.pdf

[145] Burks SV, Anderson JE, Panda B, Haider HS, Haider R, Shi D, et al. The pre-registry commercial driver medical examination: Screening sensitivity and certification lengths for two safety-related medical conditions. Journal of Occupational and Environmental Medicine. 2020;**62**(3):237-245

[146] Das AM, Chang JL, Berneking M, et al. Enhancing public health and safety by diagnosing and treating obstructive sleep apnea in the transportation industry: An American Academy of sleep medicine position statement. Journal of Clinical Sleep Medicine. 2022;**18**(10):2467-2470

[147] Mabry JE, Glenn TL, Soccolich S, Hickman JS, Durmer J. Safety benefits of a carrier-implemented sleep Apnea program for commercial motor vehicle drivers. National Surface Transportation Safety Center for Excellence report #22-UI-111. 2022. Available from: https://vtechworks.lib.vt.edu/items/dafe3979-f948-45c5-9e5e-3024833ca0b8

[148] European Union. Commission Directive 2014/85/EU of 1 July 2014, amending Directive 2006/126/EC of the European Parliament and of the Council on driving licences. OJ L 194, 2.7.2014. pp. 10-13

[149] McNicholas WT. New standards and guidelines for drivers with obstructive sleep apnea syndrome-report of the obstructive sleep apnea working group European Commission. Directorate-General for Energy and Transport. 2013. Available from: https://www.lenus.ie/bitstream/handle/10147/639197/EU_sleep_apnoea.pdf?sequence=1

[150] Schwartz DA, Vinnikov D, Blanc PD. Occupation and obstructive sleep apnea: A meta-analysis. Journal of Occupational and Environmental Medicine. 2017;**59**(6):502-508. DOI: 10.1097/JOM.0000000000001008. Erratum in: J Occup Environ Med. 2018 Jan;60(1):e74. doi: 10.1097/JOM.0000000000001219

[151] Huang G, Lee TY, Banda KJ, Pien LC, Jen HJ, Chen R, et al. Prevalence of sleep disorders among first responders for medical emergencies: A meta-analysis. Journal of Global Health. 2022;**12**:04092. DOI: 10.7189/jogh.12.04092

[152] Celikhisar H, Dasdemir IG. The association of obstructive sleep apnea syndrome and accident risk in heavy equipment operators. Medicina. 2019;**55**(9):599

[153] Aljurf TM, Olaish AH, BaHammam AS. Assessment of sleepiness, fatigue, and depression among gulf cooperation council commercial airline pilots. Sleep and Breathing. 2018;**22**:411-419

[154] Alhejaili F, Hafez A, Wali S, Alshumrani R, Alzehairi AM, Balkhyour M, et al. Prevalence of obstructive sleep Apnea among Saudi pilots. Nature and Science of Sleep. 2021;**13**:537-545. DOI: 10.2147/NSS.S299382

[155] McKay MP. Fatal consequences: Obstructive sleep apnea in a train engineer. The Annals of Family Medicine. 2015;**13**(6):583-586

[156] Koyama RG, Esteves AM, Oliveira e Silva L, Lira FS, Bittencourt LR, et al. Prevalence of and risk factors for obstructive sleep apnea syndrome in Brazilian railroad workers. Sleep Medicine. 2012;**13**:1028-1032

[157] Colquhoun CP, Casolin A. Impact of rail medical standard on obstructive sleep apnoea prevalence. Occupational medicine. 2016;**66**(1):62-68

[158] Moore BA, Tison LM, Palacios JG, Peterson AL, Mysliwiec V. Incidence of insomnia and obstructive sleep apnea in active duty United States military service members. Sleep. 2021;**44**(7):zsab024

[159] Mysliwiec V, Brock MS, Pruiksma KE, Straud CL, Taylor DJ, Hansen S, et al. A comprehensive evaluation of insomnia, obstructive sleep apnea and comorbid insomnia and obstructive sleep apnea in US military personnel. Sleep. 2022;**45**(12):zsac203. DOI: 10.1093/sleep/zsac203

[160] Goldie C, Stork B, Bernhardt K, Gaydos SJ, Kelley AM. Obstructive sleep apnea among Army aircrew. Aerospace Medicine and Human Performance. 2022;**93**(5):415-420

[161] Mysliwiec V, Martin JL, Ulmer CS, Chowdhuri S, Brock MS, Spevak C, et al. The Management of Chronic Insomnia Disorder and Obstructive Sleep Apnea: Synopsis of the 2019 U.S. Department of Veterans Affairs and U.S. Department of Defense clinical practice guidelines. Annals of Internal Medicine. 2020;**172**(5):325-336. DOI: 10.7326/M19-3575. Epub 2020 Feb 18. Erratum in: Ann Intern Med. 2021 Apr;174(4):584. doi: 10.7326/L20-1419

Chapter 6

The Influence of Risk Perception on Hearing Conservation and the Use of Hearing Protection Devices

Zhaleh Sedghi Noushabadi

Abstract

Occupational noise exposure is a pervasive hazard that continues to affect millions of workers globally, contributing significantly to noise-induced hearing loss (NIHL). Despite advancements in engineering controls and personal protective equipment, the prevalence of occupational hearing loss remains a critical concern. This paper explores the relationship between risk perception and hearing conservation behaviors, particularly the use of hearing protection devices (HPDs). It examines how individual, environmental, and organizational factors influence workers' perception of noise risks and their subsequent protective behaviors. Empirical studies across various industries reveal a positive correlation between heightened risk perception and increased HPD usage, although this relationship is mediated by factors such as comfort, accessibility, and organizational support. The findings underscore the need for comprehensive education, improved HPD comfort, and a supportive safety culture to enhance risk perception and promote effective hearing conservation. Future research should focus on longitudinal studies, objective measures of HPD use, and the integration of emerging technologies to further understand and mitigate occupational hearing loss.

Keywords: risk perception, hearing protection devices, noise-induced hearing loss, safety culture, hearing conservation, occupational noise exposure

1. Introduction

Occupational noise exposure remains one of the most pervasive and challenging workplace hazards, affecting millions of workers across diverse industries worldwide. The insidious nature of noise-induced hearing loss (NIHL), coupled with its irreversible progression, underscores the critical importance of effective hearing conservation programs in noisy work environments. Despite significant advancements in engineering controls and the availability of personal protective equipment, the prevalence of occupational hearing loss continues to be a major concern for occupational health and safety professionals.

 IntechOpen

1.1 Importance of hearing protection in noisy work environments

The World Health Organization estimates that approximately 466 million people globally suffer from disabling hearing loss, with a significant proportion attributable to occupational noise exposure [1]. In the United States alone, the National Institute for Occupational Safety and Health (NIOSH) reports that about 22 million workers are exposed to hazardous noise levels annually [2]. These statistics underscore the urgent need for effective interventions to protect workers' hearing health.

The consequences of occupational hearing loss extend far beyond the individual worker, impacting various aspects of personal, professional, and societal domains:

- Reduced quality of life due to communication difficulties and social isolation
- Increased risk of workplace accidents and injuries
- Decreased work efficiency and productivity
- Substantial economic burden on healthcare systems and employers

Given these far-reaching implications, the implementation of robust hearing conservation programs is not merely a regulatory requirement but a fundamental ethical obligation for employers.

1.2 Challenges in the use of hearing protection devices by employees

While hearing protection devices (HPDs) are a critical component of hearing conservation programs, their effectiveness is largely dependent on consistent and proper use by employees. However, numerous challenges hinder the optimal utilization of HPDs in occupational settings:

- Physical discomfort, especially during prolonged use [3]
- Interference with communication and job performance
- Perceived reduction in situational awareness
- Lack of proper training on selection, fitting, and use of HPDs
- Organizational culture and social norms that do not prioritize safety

A study by Reddy et al. found that comfort was a significant predictor of HPD usage, with workers more likely to use devices they perceived as comfortable [4]. Additionally, the perception that HPDs interfere with job performance can outweigh the perceived benefits of hearing protection, leading to inconsistent use.

1.3 Role of risk perception in hearing conservation behaviors

Risk perception plays a pivotal role in shaping workers' attitudes and behaviors toward hearing protection. It refers to the subjective judgment that individuals make about the characteristics and severity of a risk. In the context of hearing conservation,

DOI: http://dx.doi.org/10.5772/intechopen.1007120

understanding how workers perceive the risks associated with noise exposure is crucial for developing effective strategies to promote HPD use and foster a culture of hearing safety.

Research has shown that risk perception is a significant predictor of protective behaviors, including the use of HPDs. A study by Vosoughi et al. found a strong positive correlation between risk perception and safety behavior adoption related to hearing conservation ($r = 0.912$, $P < 0.001$) [5]. This suggests that workers who perceive a higher risk of hearing loss are more likely to engage in protective behaviors, such as consistent HPD use.

However, the relationship between risk perception and protective behaviors is complex and influenced by various factors, including individual characteristics, environmental conditions, and organizational support. Understanding these nuances is essential for developing targeted interventions to promote hearing conservation behaviors.

2. Risk perception and hearing conservation behaviors

2.1 Definition of risk perception and influencing factors

Risk perception, in the context of occupational health and safety, refers to the subjective assessment individuals make about the potential hazards in their work environment and the likelihood of experiencing adverse health effects. In hearing conservation, risk perception encompasses workers' judgments about the dangers of noise exposure and their susceptibility to hearing loss.

Several factors influence risk perception in the context of hearing conservation:

1. Personal experience: Workers who have experienced hearing loss or know colleagues affected by it are likely to have a heightened perception of risk [6–8]

2. Knowledge and awareness: The level of understanding about the mechanisms of hearing loss and the long-term consequences of noise exposure can significantly impact risk perception [9–15].

3. Cultural and social norms: Workplace culture and peer attitudes toward safety practices can shape individual risk perceptions [16, 17].

4. Visibility of the hazard: Unlike many other occupational hazards, NIHL develops gradually, making the risk less tangible and potentially underestimated [5, 18].

5. Trust in information sources: The credibility of safety information provided by employers or health professionals can influence how workers perceive risks [19].

2.2 Psychological theories on risk perception

Several psychological theories provide frameworks for understanding risk perception and its influence on protective behaviors in hearing conservation:

1. Health belief model (HBM): This model posits that individuals are more likely to adopt protective behaviors if they perceive a threat to their health as serious and

believe that the benefits of taking action outweigh the barriers. In the context of hearing conservation, workers who perceive NIHL as a severe threat and believe in the efficacy of HPDs are more likely to use them consistently.

2. Theory of planned behavior (TPB): This theory suggests that behavioral intentions are influenced by attitudes toward the behavior, subjective norms, and perceived behavioral control. Applied to HPD use, workers are more likely to use hearing protection if they have positive attitudes toward it, perceive social support for its use, and believe they can effectively use the devices.

3. Protection motivation theory (PMT): This theory proposes that the motivation to protect oneself from health threats is influenced by threat appraisal (perceived severity and vulnerability) and coping appraisal (response efficacy and self-efficacy). In hearing conservation, workers who perceive a high threat from noise exposure and believe in their ability to use HPDs effectively are more likely to engage in protective behaviors.

2.3 Relationship between risk perception and hearing protection behaviors

The relationship between risk perception and hearing protection behaviors is complex and multifaceted. Research has consistently shown a positive correlation between higher levels of risk perception and increased use of HPDs. For instance, a study by Arezes and Miguel [9] found that workers' individual risk perception was one of the main predictors of HPD use.

However, the strength of this relationship can vary depending on various factors:

1. Accuracy of risk perception: Workers may misjudge the actual level of risk they face. A study by Svensson et al. [20] found that workers often underestimated their noise exposure levels, leading to inadequate protective behaviors.

2. Competing priorities: Even when risk is perceived accurately, other factors such as comfort, communication needs, or job demands may override the motivation to use HPDs.

3. Self-efficacy: Workers' confidence in their ability to use HPDs correctly can mediate the relationship between risk perception and protective behaviors [21].

4. Organizational support: The extent to which the workplace environment supports and encourages HPD use can strengthen or weaken the link between risk perception and behavior.

Table 1 illustrates risk perception and hearing conservation behaviors.

Understanding these nuances is crucial for developing effective interventions to promote hearing conservation behaviors. While enhancing risk perception is important, it must be coupled with strategies that address other barriers to HPD use and create a supportive environment for hearing protection.

Section	Key points
Influencing factors	1. Personal experience: Previous hearing loss or knowledge of affected colleague's increases risk perception. 2. Knowledge and awareness: Understanding hearing loss mechanisms impacts risk perception. 3. Cultural norms: Workplace culture shapes perceptions. 4. Visibility of hazard: Gradual development of NIHL makes it less tangible. 5. Trust in information: Credibility of safety information affects perception.
Psychological theories	1. Health belief model (HBM): Perception of serious health threat increases protective behaviors. 2. Theory of planned behavior (TPB): Intentions influenced by attitudes, norms, and perceived control. 3. Protection motivation theory (PMT): Motivation based on threat appraisal and coping appraisal.
Relationship between risk perception and hearing protection behaviors	Positive correlation between risk perception and HPD use. Factors affecting this relationship: 1. Accuracy of risk perception: Misjudgment can lead to inadequate protection. 2. Competing priorities: Comfort and job demands may override motivation. 3. Self-efficacy: Confidence in using HPDs influences behavior. 4. Organizational support: Workplace support can strengthen or weaken the behavior link.

Table 1.
Risk perception and hearing conservation behaviors.

3. Factors influencing risk perception in hearing conservation

3.1 Individual characteristics

Individual characteristics play a significant role in shaping risk perception related to hearing conservation. These factors can influence how workers interpret and respond to information about noise hazards and the importance of hearing protection.

1. Age: Age has been found to have a complex relationship with risk perception in hearing conservation. Older workers may have a heightened perception of risk due to accumulated experience or personal encounters with hearing loss. Conversely, they may also exhibit a form of risk habituation if they have worked in noisy environments for extended periods without apparent consequences. A study by Reddy et al. [4] found that older workers were more likely to use HPDs consistently, suggesting a possible link between age and risk perception.

2. Gender: Research has indicated that gender can influence risk perception and subsequent protective behaviors. For instance, Svensson et al. [20] observed that female workers in industrial settings were more likely to report higher levels of

perceived risk from noise exposure compared to their male counterparts. This difference in risk perception may be attributed to various factors, including socialization patterns and general health awareness.

3. Work experience: The length of time an individual has worked in noisy environments can affect their risk perception. Workers with more experience may have a more accurate understanding of noise hazards, but they may also develop a sense of invulnerability if they have not experienced noticeable hearing loss. Vosoughi et al. found that workers with longer job tenure had higher levels of risk perception regarding hearing conservation [5].

4. Education and training: The level of education and specific training in hearing conservation can significantly impact risk perception. Workers who have received comprehensive education about the mechanisms of hearing loss and the importance of protection are likely to have a more accurate perception of risk. Lie et al. [22] demonstrated that targeted educational interventions could enhance risk perception and improve HPD usage rates.

3.2 Environmental factors

Environmental factors in the workplace can significantly influence workers' perception of noise-related risks and their motivation to use HPDs.

1. Noise levels: The intensity and duration of noise exposure are critical factors in shaping risk perception. Paradoxically, extremely high noise levels may lead to desensitization, potentially reducing perceived risk. Conversely, moderate but consistent noise levels might maintain a heightened sense of risk. Arezes and Miguel [9] found that workers' perception of noise levels did not always align with actual measured levels, highlighting the subjective nature of risk perception.

2. Visibility of hazard: Unlike many other occupational hazards, noise is invisible, and its effects are often gradual. This lack of immediate, visible consequences can lead to underestimation of risk. Strategies that make the hazard more tangible, such as noise level indicators or regular audiometric testing, can enhance risk perception.

3. Accessibility of HPDs: The availability and ease of access to HPDs can influence risk perception. When HPDs are readily available and their use is facilitated by the work environment, workers may perceive a higher level of organizational commitment to safety, potentially enhancing their own risk awareness [23].

3.3 Organizational factors

Organizational factors play a crucial role in shaping the context within which workers form their perceptions of risk and make decisions about hearing protection.

1. Safety culture: The overall safety culture of an organization significantly influences individual risk perceptions. In workplaces where safety is visibly prioritized and consistently enforced, workers are more likely to have heightened risk

awareness. Reddy et al. found that a strong safety culture was positively associated with higher risk perception and increased HPD use [4].

2. Management support: The level of support and commitment from management toward hearing conservation efforts can greatly impact workers' risk perceptions. When management actively promotes and participates in hearing protection initiatives, it sends a strong signal about the importance of the issue, potentially elevating risk perception among workers.

3. Communication strategies: The way information about noise hazards and hearing protection is communicated within the organization can influence risk perception. Clear, consistent, and engaging communication strategies can enhance understanding and awareness of risks.

4. Peer influence: The attitudes and behaviors of coworkers can significantly shape an individual's risk perception. In environments where HPD use is normalized and valued among peers, individual workers are more likely to perceive higher levels of risk and engage in protective behaviors.

5. Regulatory compliance: The extent to which an organization adheres to and goes beyond regulatory requirements for hearing conservation can impact workers' risk perceptions. Strict compliance and proactive measures can reinforce the seriousness of noise hazards.

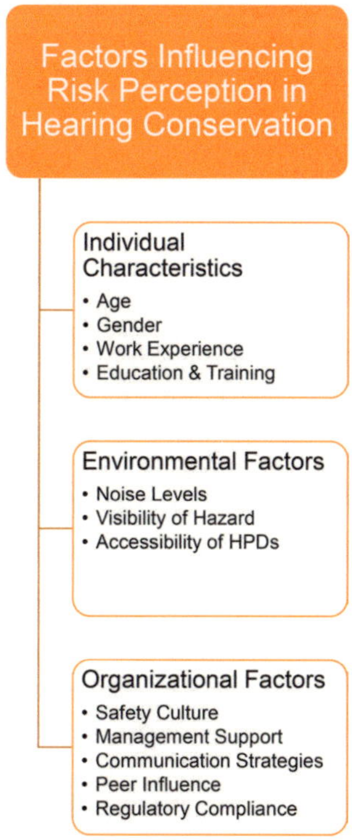

Figure 1.
Factors influencing risk perception in hearing conservation.

Figure 1 illustrates the factors influencing risk perception in hearing conservation.

Understanding these multifaceted influences on risk perception is crucial for developing comprehensive and effective hearing conservation programs. By addressing individual, environmental, and organizational factors, occupational health and safety professionals can create strategies that not only enhance risk perception but also translate this awareness into consistent protective behaviors.

4. Empirical studies on risk perception and hearing conservation

4.1 Review of studies in various industrial and occupational settings

Empirical research on risk perception and hearing conservation has been conducted across a wide range of industrial and occupational settings, providing valuable insights into the complex relationship between perceived risk and protective behaviors.

1. Manufacturing industry: A study by Arezes and Miguel [9] in Portuguese manufacturing plants examined the factors influencing HPD use among 516 workers. The study found that individual risk perception was one of the main predictors of HPD use, along with the perceived value of hearing preservation. Importantly, the study highlighted that workers' perceptions of noise levels often differed from actual measured levels, emphasizing the subjective nature of risk assessment.

2. Construction sector: Svensson et al. [20] investigated risk perception and HPD use among construction workers in Sweden. The study revealed that while most workers were aware of the risks associated with noise exposure, there was a significant discrepancy between perceived and actual noise levels. This misalignment in risk perception led to inadequate use of hearing protection, especially in situations where noise levels were underestimated.

3. Healthcare settings: Although not typically associated with high noise levels, certain healthcare environments can pose risks to hearing. Rawool and Campbell [24] conducted a study among healthcare workers exposed to noise from medical equipment. The research found that risk perception varied significantly based on job roles and prior education about noise hazards. Notably, workers who had received specific training on the risks of noise exposure in healthcare settings demonstrated higher levels of risk awareness and were more likely to use HPDs when necessary.

4. Mining industry: A comprehensive study by Bockstael et al. [25] in the mining sector examined the relationship between noise exposure, risk perception, and HPD use. The study found a strong correlation between perceived risk and the likelihood of using hearing protection. However, it also highlighted that risk perception alone was not sufficient to ensure consistent HPD use, emphasizing the need for complementary strategies such as improving HPD comfort and accessibility.
   A comprehensive study by Liebenberg et al. [26] examined the impact of noise exposure on miners in the mining sector. The findings revealed that nearly 60% of miners reported experiencing high noise exposure for over 10 years, leading

to hearing issues such as tinnitus. While 71% of participants believed that their workplace noise control strategies were effective, this primarily pertained to the use of HPDs. The study also identified a significant gap in the urgency of risk management for NIHL, despite the awareness of its long-term consequences, indicating the need for more proactive measures in addressing these risks.

5. Agriculture: Cramer et al. [27] investigated risk perception and hearing protection behaviors among agricultural workers. The study revealed unique challenges in this sector, including the intermittent nature of noise exposure and the influence of traditional practices. Risk perception was found to be lower compared to other industrial sectors, partly due to the lack of consistent noise exposure and limited access to occupational health services.

6. Printing industry: A study by Vosoughi et al. [5] investigated the relationship between risk perception and the use of HPDs among printing workers. The findings revealed a significant positive correlation between risk perception and the adoption of safety behaviors, with a p-value of less than 0.001. Workers who had higher levels of risk perception regarding noise exposure were more likely to utilize HPDs, indicated by a correlation coefficient of $r_s = 0.912$ ($P < 0.001$). However, it was notable that only 28.9% of participants consistently used HPDs, highlighting a critical gap between awareness of the risks and actual protective practices in the workplace.

A study by Basheer et al. [28] examined the awareness and attitudes of printing press workers regarding NIHL. The findings indicated that these workers had inadequate knowledge about NIHL, reflected in a mean knowledge score of only 55.6%. Despite over 80% acknowledging that excessive noise could result in permanent hearing loss, many exhibited negative attitudes toward preventive measures. Notably, a significant majority (70%) reported never having used ear protection devices, underscoring a critical area for intervention to enhance hearing safety in the printing industry.

4.2 Findings on the relationship between risk perception and HPD use

Across these diverse studies, several consistent findings emerge regarding the relationship between risk perception and the use of HPDs:

1. Positive correlation: Most studies report a positive correlation between higher levels of risk perception and increased likelihood of HPD use. For instance, Vosoughi et al. found a strong positive correlation ($r = 0.912$, $P < 0.001$) between risk perception and safety behavior adoption related to hearing conservation [5].

2. Mediating factors: While risk perception is important, its influence on HPD use is often mediated by other factors. These include the perceived effectiveness of HPDs, comfort and ease of use, and organizational support for hearing conservation practices [29–31].

3. Accuracy of risk perception: Several studies highlight discrepancies between perceived and actual noise exposure levels. This misalignment can lead to inadequate protection even when general awareness of risks is high [32].

4. Influence of training: Studies consistently show that targeted education and training can enhance risk perception and improve HPD usage rates. However, the long-term effectiveness of training interventions varies, suggesting the need for ongoing reinforcement [33–39].

5. Sector-specific variations: The strength of the relationship between risk perception and HPD use varies across different industrial sectors, influenced by factors such as the nature of noise exposure, workplace culture, and regulatory environments [40].

4.3 Challenges and limitations of previous studies

Despite the valuable insights gained from empirical studies on risk perception and hearing conservation, several challenges and limitations persist:

1. Methodological limitations: Many studies rely on cross-sectional designs, which provide a snapshot of risk perception and HPD use at a single point in time. This limits the ability to draw causal conclusions about the relationship between these variables. Longitudinal studies are needed to better understand how risk perception evolves over time and its impact on protective behaviors.

2. Self-reported data: A significant portion of research relies on self-reported data regarding HPD use and risk perception. This can introduce bias, as individuals may overestimate their adherence to safety practices or misreport their perceptions of risk. Objective measures, such as direct observations or audiometric testing, could enhance the reliability of findings.

3. Generalizability: Many studies focus on specific industries or geographic locations, which may limit the generalizability of findings to other contexts. Further research is needed across diverse occupational settings to develop a more comprehensive understanding of risk perception and hearing conservation.

4. Complex interactions: The interplay between individual, environmental, and organizational factors influencing risk perception is complex and multifaceted. Future research should explore these interactions in greater depth to identify effective intervention strategies.

5. Cultural context: Risk perception is influenced by cultural factors that may not be adequately addressed in existing studies. Understanding how cultural beliefs and values shape perceptions of noise hazards and protective behaviors is essential for designing culturally relevant interventions.

5. Strategies to enhance risk perception and improve hearing conservation behaviors

5.1 Education and awareness raising

One of the most effective strategies for enhancing risk perception is through comprehensive education and awareness-raising initiatives. These can include:

1. Comprehensive training programs: Implementing in-depth training sessions that educate workers about the risks of noise exposure, the mechanisms of hearing loss, and the importance of HPDs can significantly improve risk perception and protective behaviors. These programs should be tailored to the specific work environment and include both theoretical knowledge and practical skills [41]. For example, Lie et al. [22] demonstrated that targeted educational interventions could enhance risk perception and improve HPD usage rates.

2. Interactive workshops: Organizing interactive workshops that involve hands-on practice with HPDs can enhance understanding and comfort. These sessions can include demonstrations of proper HPD usage, discussions about the long-term consequences of noise exposure, and opportunities for workers to ask questions and share experiences.

3. Regular auditory testing: Implementing regular audiometric testing and providing feedback on hearing status can create a sense of urgency regarding hearing protection. When workers receive information about their hearing health, they may be more motivated to use HPDs consistently. Rawool and Campbell [24] found that workers who had received specific information about their hearing status demonstrated higher levels of risk awareness.

4. Visual aids and signage: Utilizing visual aids, such as posters, infographics, and digital displays, can effectively communicate the risks associated with noise exposure and the benefits of HPDs. Clear and engaging visuals can enhance understanding and retention of information, making it easier for workers to grasp the importance of hearing conservation.

5. Peer education programs: Implementing peer-led education initiatives can be particularly effective in enhancing risk perception. Workers may be more receptive to information and advice from colleagues who have similar experiences and understand the specific challenges of their work environment.

5.2 Improving access and comfort of HPDs

Enhancing the accessibility and comfort of HPDs can significantly improve their usage:

1. Variety of options: Providing a range of HPD options can help accommodate different preferences and comfort levels. This may include various types of earplugs (foam, pre-molded, custom-molded) and earmuffs. A study by Reddy et al. [4] found that comfort was a significant predictor of HPD usage.

2. Custom-fitted devices: Offering custom-fitted HPDs can improve comfort and effectiveness. These devices are tailored to the individual's ear canal shape, potentially increasing both comfort and protection.

3. Ease of use: Ensuring that HPDs are easy to use and maintain can encourage consistent usage. This includes providing clear instructions, demonstrations on proper insertion and removal techniques, and guidance on maintenance and replacement schedules.

4. Accessibility: Making HPDs readily available at multiple locations throughout the workplace can increase their use. This might involve installing dispensers at entrances to noisy areas or providing personal carrying cases for workers.

5. Integration with other PPE: For workplaces where multiple types of personal protective equipment (PPE) are required, integrating HPDs with other equipment (e.g., hard hats with attached earmuffs) can improve convenience and consistency of use.

5.3 Creating a supportive organizational environment

Developing a supportive organizational culture is crucial for enhancing risk perception and promoting consistent HPD use:

1. Management engagement: Active involvement of management in promoting hearing conservation can significantly influence workers' attitudes toward HPDs. This can include regular communication about the importance of hearing protection, participation in training sessions, and visible use of HPDs by managers when in noisy areas.

2. Safety culture development: Fostering a strong safety culture that prioritizes hearing conservation can enhance overall risk perception. This involves integrating hearing protection into broader safety initiatives and consistently reinforcing its importance.

3. Incentive programs: Implementing well-designed incentive programs that reward safe behaviors, including consistent HPD usage, can motivate workers to prioritize hearing protection. However, care should be taken to ensure that such programs do not inadvertently discourage reporting of hearing issues or near-misses.

4. Regular monitoring and feedback: Implementing systems for regular monitoring of noise levels and HPD use, coupled with constructive feedback to workers, can reinforce the importance of hearing protection and help identify areas for improvement.

5. Open communication channels: Establishing clear channels for workers to report concerns about noise levels or difficulties with HPD use can help address issues promptly and demonstrate organizational commitment to hearing health.

6. Discussion

Recent publications in the field of occupational health have emphasized the pressing need for enhanced strategies to address NIHL and improve the effectiveness of hearing conservation programs. For instance, studies have increasingly focused on the role of risk perception in influencing protective behaviors, highlighting that a worker's understanding of the risks associated with noise exposure is pivotal in determining their use of HPDs. Vosoughi et al. [5] demonstrated a strong correlation between risk perception and safety behavior adoption, reinforcing the idea that increasing awareness can lead to more consistent HPD usage.

Moreover, recent research has expanded on the psychological theories of risk perception, such as the Health Belief Model and the Theory of Planned Behavior, to better understand how individual attitudes and social norms affect protective behaviors. These insights are crucial as they suggest that interventions aimed at modifying risk perception should not only focus on imparting knowledge but also on fostering a culture of safety within organizations.

However, despite the growing body of evidence supporting the importance of risk perception, challenges remain. Many workers still demonstrate a disconnect between their awareness of noise hazards and their actual protective practices. This gap indicates that simply increasing knowledge may not be sufficient; practical barriers, such as discomfort with HPDs and workplace culture, must also be addressed.

To enhance the quality and impact of future research, it is essential to adopt a more holistic approach that not only encompasses individual and organizational factors but also considers the broader sociocultural context in which workers operate. For example, integrating qualitative methods, such as interviews and focus groups, could provide deeper insights into the lived experiences of workers regarding noise exposure and HPD use.

Additionally, exploring innovative technologies, such as wearable devices that monitor noise exposure in real-time, could offer new avenues for enhancing risk perception and promoting safer behaviors. By combining these approaches, future studies can contribute to a more comprehensive understanding of how to effectively mitigate the risks of NIHL and promote a culture of hearing conservation across various industries.

7. Conclusion and future recommendations

7.1 Summary of key findings

This chapter has explored the complex relationship between risk perception and hearing conservation behaviors, particularly focusing on the use of HPDs in occupational settings. Key findings include:

1. Risk perception plays a crucial role in shaping workers' attitudes and behaviors toward hearing protection, with higher levels of perceived risk generally associated with increased HPD use.

2. Multiple factors influence risk perception, including individual characteristics (age, gender, work experience, education), environmental factors (noise levels, visibility of hazard), and organizational factors (safety culture, management support).

3. Psychological theories such as the Health Belief Model, Theory of Planned Behavior, and Protection Motivation Theory provide valuable frameworks for understanding the relationship between risk perception and protective behaviors.

4. Empirical studies across various industries consistently show a positive correlation between risk perception and HPD use, as well as highlight the complexity of this relationship and the influence of mediating factors.

5. Effective strategies to enhance risk perception and improve hearing conservation behaviors include comprehensive education and awareness programs, improving HPD accessibility and comfort, and creating a supportive organizational environment.

7.2 Limitations and future research directions

While significant progress has been made in understanding the role of risk perception in hearing conservation, several limitations and areas for future research remain:

1. Longitudinal studies: Most existing research relies on cross-sectional data. Future studies should employ longitudinal designs to better understand how risk perception evolves over time and its long-term impact on protective behaviors.

2. Objective measures: There is a need for more studies that incorporate objective measures of HPD use and noise exposure, rather than relying solely on self-reported data.

3. Cultural and contextual factors: Further research is needed to explore how cultural differences and specific work contexts influence risk perception and hearing conservation behaviors.

4. Intervention effectiveness: More rigorous evaluation of intervention strategies is required to determine the most effective approaches for enhancing risk perception and promoting consistent HPD use across different occupational settings.

5. Technology integration: Future research should explore the potential of emerging technologies (e.g., smart HPDs, mobile apps for noise monitoring) in enhancing risk perception and facilitating hearing protection behaviors.

6. Holistic approach: Studies that examine hearing conservation within the broader context of overall occupational health and safety may provide valuable insights into integrated approaches to risk management.

By addressing these research gaps and continuing to refine our understanding of the relationship between risk perception and hearing conservation behaviors, we can develop more effective strategies to protect workers' hearing health and reduce the global burden of occupational NIHL.

Acknowledgements

In this section, I would like to express my heartfelt gratitude to my esteemed mentor, Prof. Shahram Vosoughi, a faculty member of the Department of Occupational Health Engineering at Iran University of Medical Sciences, for his invaluable support and encouragement in writing this chapter. His guidance and expertise have greatly contributed to my understanding and the overall quality of this work.

Author details

Zhaleh Sedghi Noushabadi
Occupational Health Engineering Department, School of Public Health, Iran University of Medical Sciences (IUMS), Tehran, Iran

*Address all correspondence to: zhaleh.sedghy@gmail.com

References

[1] Organization World Health. Deafness and Hearing Loss. 2024. Available from: https://www.who.int/news-room/fact-sheets/detail/deafness-and-hearing-loss

[2] National Institute for Occupational Safety and Health (NIOSH). Occupational Hearing Loss Surveillance. 2024. Available from: https://www.cdc.gov/niosh/noise/surveillance/index.html

[3] Muda WM, Maamor N, Wahat NH. Noise exposure level among shopping mall workers in Kuala Lumpur. International Journal of Allied Health Sciences. 2019;**3**(1):559. DOI: 10.31436/ijahs.v3i1.228

[4] Reddy RK, Welch D, Thorne P, Ameratunga S. Hearing protection use in manufacturing workers: A qualitative study. Journal of Noise and Health. 2012;**14**(59):202-209. DOI: 10.4103/1463-1741.99896

[5] Vosoughi S, Alimohammadi I, Hosseini AF, Sedghi Noushabadi Z. Relationship between risk perception toward hearing conservation and using hearing protection devices among offset printing workers in Tehran province, Iran. Archives of Environmental Occupational Health. 2022;**77**(4):338-344. DOI: 10.1080/19338244.2021.1893630

[6] Fauzan NS, Sukadarin EH, Widia M, Irianto I, Ghazali I. A systematic literature review of the factors influencing hearing protection device usage among industrial workers. International Journal of Environmental Research Public Health. 2023;**20**(4):2934. DOI: 10.3390/ijerph20042934

[7] AlYahya KA, Alarfaj AA, Al-Zahir BZ, AlMulhim DA, Al Hussain RS, Alfalah RR, et al. Awareness of noise-induced hearing loss among the general population in the Eastern Province of Saudi Arabia. Saudi Journal of Otorhinolaryngology Head and Neck Surgery. 1 Oct 2023;**25**(4):188-205. DOI: 10.4103/sjoh.sjoh_59_22

[8] Ilyas M, Othmani A, Nait-Ali A. Computer-aided prediction of hearing loss based on auditory perception. Multimedia Tools and Applications. 2020;**79**:15765-15789. DOI: 10.1007/s11042-020-08910-w

[9] Arezes PM, Miguel A. Risk perception and safety behaviour: A study in an occupational environment. Journal of Safety Science. 2008;**46**(6):900-907. DOI: 10.1016/j.ssci.2007.11.008

[10] Vosoughi S, Alimohammadi I, Hosseini AF, Noushabadi Z. Case study: Knowledge, attitude, and practice (KAP) regarding hearing protection: A case study among offset printing industry workers in Tehran province. Noise Control Engineering Journal. 2022;**70**(3):270-278. DOI: 10.3397/1/377021

[11] Vosoughi S, Alimohammadi I, Hosseini AF, Sedghi Z. Designing a questionnaire to investigate the knowledge, attitude, and practice (KAP) of printing industry workers regarding hearing protection and determining its validity and reliability. Journal of Occupational Hygiene Engineering. 2019;**6**(1):43-51. DOI: 10.21859/johe.6.1.6

[12] Ishak NA, Fauzan NS, Widia M. Correlation between noise-related risk perception, knowledge and the use of hearing protection device: A case study among landfill workers. In: American Institute of Physics Conference Series. Vol. 2682. No. 1. AIP Publishing; Feb 2023. p. 060010. DOI: 10.1063/5.0114277

[13] Ata Teneler A, Hassoy H. Evaluation of risk perception related with environmental noise among residents living in different vicinities of wind turbines. International Journal of Environmental Health Research. 2024;**34**(3):1788-1799. DOI: 10.1080/09603123.2023.2245344

[14] Washnik NJ, Russell JA, Bhatt I, Meier R, Chuzie O, Nadeau N, et al. University marching band members' noise dosages and hearing health-related knowledge. International Journal of Environmental Research and Public Health. 2021;**18**(21):11497. DOI: 10.3390/ijerph182111497

[15] Yévenes-Briones H, Carrasco-Alarcón P, Sanhueza H, Acevedo N, Venturelli R, Morales C. Chilean dentists' knowledge of hearing loss generated by occupational noise exposure. Revista de la Facultad de Medicina. 2021;**69**(2):e79902. DOI: 10.15446/revfacmed.v69n2.79902

[16] Arezes PM, Miguel A. Hearing protection use in industry: The role of risk perception. Jounral of Safety Science. 2005;**43**(4):253-267. DOI: 10.1016/j.ssci.2005.07.002

[17] Ibili F, Adams CA, Adebanji AO, Andam-Akorful SA. The state-of-the-art of practice of traffic noise regulations in Ghana. Noise & Vibration Worldwide. 2023;**54**(4-5):204-214. DOI: 10.1177/09574565231161645

[18] Millet B, Snapp HA, Rajguru SM, Schaefer SN. Prevalence of hearing loss and perceptions of hearing health and protection among Florida firefighters. International Journal of Environmental Research and Public Health. 2023;**20**(5):3826. DOI: 10.3390/ijerph20053826

[19] Broyles G, Kardous CA, Shaw PB, Krieg EF. Noise exposures and perceptions of hearing conservation programs among wildland firefighters. Journal of Occupational and Environmental Hygiene. 2019;**16**(12):775-784. DOI: 10.1080/15459624.2019.1668001

[20] Svensson EB, Morata TC, Nylén P, Krieg EF, Johnson A-C. Beliefs and attitudes among Swedish workers regarding the risk of hearing loss. International Journal of Audiology. 2004;**43**(10):585-593. DOI: 10.1080/14992020400050075

[21] Nelson NL, Killion MC, Lentz JJ, Kidd GR. Hearing protection success: Musicians have a favorable response to hearing protection and listeners are unable to identify music produced by musicians wearing hearing protection. Journal of the American Academy of Audiology. 2020;**31**(10):763-770. DOI: 10.1055/s-0040-1719128

[22] Lie A, Skogstad M, Johannessen HA, Tynes T, Mehlum IS, Nordby K-C, et al. Occupational noise exposure and hearing: A systematic review. International Archives of Occupational Environmental Health. 2016;**89**:351-372. DOI: 10.1007/s00420-015-1083-5

[23] Giliberti C, Castro FL, Orlando MP, Mariconte R, Diano M. Use of hearing aids at work: Results of a questionnaire for the analysis of comfort and perceived benefit. Human Factors in Accessibility and Assistive Technology. 2022;**37**:37. DOI: 10.54941/ahfe1001640

[24] Rawool VW, Campbell C. Effectiveness of earmuffs in protecting hearing during shooting practice: A case-study. International Journal of Audiology. 2018;**57**(7):545-552. DOI: 10.1080/14992027.2018.1441556

[25] Bockstael A, De Bruyne L, Vinck B, Botteldooren D. Hearing protection in

industry: Companies' policy and workers' perception. International Journal of Industrial Ergonomics. 2013;**43**(6):512-517. DOI: 10.1016/j.ergon.2012.08.009

[26] Liebenberg A, Oosthuizen J, Reed S. A current affair: Worker perceptions of noise exposure and occupational hearing loss in Australian coal mines. Annals of Work Exposures and Health. 2023;**67**(9):1111-1120. DOI: 10.1093/annweh/wxad055

[27] Cramer ME, Wendl MJ, Sayles H, Duysen E, Achutan C. Knowledge, attitudes, and practices for respiratory and hearing health among Midwestern farmers. Public Health Nursing. 2017;**34**(4):348-358. DOI: 10.1111/phn.12306

[28] Basheer R, Bhargavi PG, Prakash HP. Knowledge, attitude, and practice of printing press workers towards noise-induced hearing loss. Noise and Health. 2019;**21**(99):62-68. DOI: 10.4103/nah.NAH_9_19

[29] McGuinn P, Buggy C, Drummond A, Sripaiboonkij P. Factors influencing the use of hearing protection devices in Irish mine workers. International Journal of Occupational and Environmental Safety. 2021;**5**(2):51-61. DOI: 10.24840/2184-0954_005.002_0005

[30] Kwak C, Han W. The effectiveness of hearing protection devices: A systematic review and meta-analysis. International Journal of Environmental Research and Public Health. 2021;**18**(21):11693. DOI: 10.3390/ijerph182111693

[31] Costa N, Abreu S, Arezes PM. Alarm detection in noise work environments: The influence of hearing protection devices. In: Safety, Reliability and Risk Analysis. CRC Press; 18 Sep 2013. pp. 1651-1655

[32] Lepcha A, Mammen MD, Augustine AM, Philip A. Audiological effects of occupational noise exposure in high-risk staff in a tertiary care hospital in South India. Annals of Otology and Neurotology. 2019;**2**(01):A003. DOI: 10.1055/s-0039-1700196

[33] Casali JG, Murphy WJ. Happy ears for many years: Selected papers from the 2018 annual conference of the National Hearing Conservation Association. International Journal of Audiology. 2019;**58**(sup1):S1-S2. DOI: 10.1080/14992027.2018.1546476

[34] Eichwald J, Scinicariello F. Survey of teen noise exposure and efforts to protect hearing at school — United States, 2020. MMWR. Morbidity and Mortality Weekly Report. 2020;**69**:1822-1826. DOI: 10.15585/mmwr.mm6948a5

[35] Morata TC, Meinke DK. An amazing 10-year collection of hearing loss prevention supplements by the National Hearing Conservation Association. International Journal of Audiology. 2020;**59**(sup1):S1-S2. DOI: 10.1080/14992027.2020.1699329

[36] Eichwald J, Themann CL, Scinicariello F. Safe listening at venues and events with amplified music — United States, 2022. MMWR. Morbidity and Mortality Weekly Report. 2023;**72**:338-341. DOI: 10.15585/mmwr.mm7213a3

[37] Mirzaei RA, Rakhshani F. Factors affecting the use of hearing protection devices among industrial workers of Sistan and Baluchestan province. The Journal of Infectious Diseases. 2012;**16**(3):66-71

[38] Jahangiri M, Mirzaei R, Ansari H. Risk perception, knowledge and safety attitude and hearing protector use in petrochemical industry workers. Audiology. 2008;**17**(1):11-18

[39] Corbett DA, Whitelaw JL. Does perception equal protection? occupational noise exposure & hearing protective device utilisation for engineering trades. In: Australian Institute of Occupational Hygienists 34th Annual Conference. 2016. pp. 43-53

[40] Degeest S, Maes L, Leyssens L, Keppler H. The test–retest reliability of questionnaires regarding attitudes and beliefs toward noise, hearing loss, and hearing protector devices in young adults. Noise and Health. 2018;**20**(93):31-36. DOI: 10.4103/nah.NAH_41_17

[41] Hong O, Samo D, Hulea R, Eakin B. Perception and attitudes of firefighters on noise exposure and hearing loss. Journal of Occupational and Environmental Hygiene. 2008;**5**(3):210-215. DOI: 10.1080/15459620701880659

Chapter 7

Predicting Pneumoconiosis and Chronic Obstructive Pulmonary Disease Risks in Coal Miners in Donbass

Olga Yurievna Nikolenko, Dmitry Olegovich Lastkov, Oleg Viktorovich Partas and Inna Sergeevna Eromyants

Abstract

The problem of dust-related respiratory diseases caused by exposure to fibrogenic aerosols remains relevant for the majority of leading economies of the world, which is associated with significant financial loss on the part of both workers and employers, including the social insurance system. To predict dust-related respiratory disease (pneumoconiosis and chronic obstructive pulmonary disease) risk, a matrix was created and distributed into three arrays in each nosology. The most effective second array included the following indices: mining geological, working conditions, age and experience characteristics; spirography indices; general analysis; and biochemical blood indices. As a result, the function of predicting disease development (pneumoconiosis or chronic obstructive pulmonary disease) was derived. The following variables were selected as predictors of this model: coal seam angle, forced vital capacity, inspiratory vital capacity, cortisol, diene conjugates, malonic dialdehyde, plasma antioxidant activity, catalase, vitamin E, uric acid, and xanthine oxidase. In all cases, $p < 0.05$. Based on the matrix classification of the analyzed sample (2/3rd of the total sample size in proportion to each disease), the effectiveness of the model in predicting disease development under study is 91.32% (pneumoconiosis—88.52% and chronic obstructive pulmonary disease—94.11%). In cross-validation (1/3rd of the total sample size in proportion to each disease), model correctness comprises 82.15% (pneumoconiosis and chronic obstructive pulmonary disease—73.13% and 91.17%, respectively).

Keywords: pneumoconiosis, chronic obstructive pulmonary disease, coal miners, Donbass, mining geological, working conditions, experience characteristics, spirography indices, general analysis, biochemical blood indices

1. Introduction

Good health of the working population is known to be the key to productive societal development. Today, it is no longer enough for modern management to be able to mobilize workers promptly and concentrate them in those production sectors that are priorities from the point of view of economic development. No less important is the problem of preserving labor potential at a qualitatively capable level, creating labor teams that are not only capable of productive work but also resistant to the impact of excessive physical and psycho-emotional stresses, and providing conditions that reduce the probability of occupational and industrial diseases. Risks of health disorders in the coal industry are much higher than in other industries.

The main harmful production factors at underground workplaces of coal enterprises include dustiness of the working zone air, which is present practically at all workplaces and varies widely. Occupational morbidity in the coal industry of Donbass is the leading among all industries [1].

In Donbass, research on the formation, spreading, and deposition of dust in the dust formation, distribution, and deposition in miners began to be intensively carried out with the introduction of high-performance equipment in the 50s of the twentieth century. The fundamental works, which determined the directions of scientific research in this field in this period, are academician A.A. Skochinsky's ones. In 1953, based on Prof. A.S. Burchakov's research results, "Guide for workers of dust ventilation service at coal mines and project organizations on the use of ventilation design organizations on the use of ventilation as a means of dust control" was published, and in 1965 Prof. A.S. Burchakov and Prof. A.I. Ksenofontova published the monograph "Theory and practice of dust control in coal mines" [2].

Respiratory diseases occupy the first place among occupational diseases in the coal industry. Occupational morbidity remains a complex hygienic and socioeconomic problem. Dust-related respiratory diseases (DRD) are accompanied by persistent disability of victims with subsequent disability [3, 4]. DRD problem caused by fibrogenic aerosol exposure remains relevant for most of the world's leading economies, which is associated with significant financial losses, both patient's and employer's, including the social insurance system [5–8].

In the conditions of modern production in various industries, the reality of exposure to a complex of unfavorable factors of labor activity (dust, noise, vibration, uncomfortable microclimate, etc.) remains. Due to their impact, the worker's functional state changes and adaptive capabilities are reduced, which leads to an increased risk of occupational diseases [9].

Dust factor in the air of the working zone, despite the actively carried out anti-dust measures, in some industries continues to remain in the category of leading unfavorable production factors. The share of occupational dust pathology in the structure of occupational morbidity in the Russian Federation is large. All these factors make it necessary to conduct research to substantiate the occupational risk for workers in dust occupations [10].

Coal-rock dust is a powerful damaging factor that causes the development of DRD in miners [11, 12]. The probability of getting an occupational disease of dust etiology depends on the following factors: (1) dust concentration, intensity of dust exposure, contact duration (work experience); (2) individual sensitivity to dust and the presence of factors predisposing to the development of fibrosis; (3) the nature of dust, geometric dimensions of particles, their aerodynamic properties [13–17]. It is important to improve continuously the assessment methodology of hygienically significant characteristics of dust exposure to specify hygienic criteria of hazard and harmfulness of working conditions by dust factor, as well as to justify more effective measures to protect the workers' health employed in dust-forming technological processes [18].

The effect of coal dust on coal miners can cause not only fibrotic process in the lungs, that is, pneumoconiosis, but also chronic obstructive pulmonary disease, emphysema, and chronic bronchitis, which do not differ from those caused by tobacco smoke. It is established that the highest concentrations of dust are observed at mining sites, and pneumoconiosis develops more often in miners working at them [19–21].

Working conditions at workplaces, labor process severity, and the structure of occupational routes affect the timing of occupational disease development in miners from dust action. In more than half of the cases (55–58%), diseases are detected at working age. Retirement terms of 20–25 years of work experience do not allow to avoid sanitary dangerous doses of dust accumulation [22–24].

It was found that before 1997, pneumoconiosis was more severe, and classical forms prevailed: silicosis and silicotuberculosis, which were characterized by more significant and early clinical, functional, and radiological changes in the lungs. In silicotuberculosis, pronounced disorders of external respiratory function (55.0%) and obstructive-restrictive type of ventilation disorders (72.0%) were registered. Nodular darkening was predominantly of 'p' type 50.0% and 'q' type 30.0% with massive fibrosis. After 1997, more benign development of pneumoconiosis was noted, and interstitial, mixed forms were more frequent. The radiological picture is mainly presented in the form of interstitial fibrosis expressed indistinctly and linear darkening of the type 's' and 's/t' [25].

In Y.Sh. Halimov's work, the clinical case of late pneumoconiosis was described. The disease developed 25 years after contact cessation with fibrogenic dust. The diagnosis was made on the basis of occupational anamnesis; sanitary and hygienic characteristics of working condition data; clinical examination results, including physical and laboratory methods; spirography; fibrobronchoscopy; radiography; and computed tomography of the lungs [26].

One of the priority areas of preventive medicine is the study of general regularities and mechanisms of the impact of industrial environmental factors, primarily dust, on humans [27]. According to their origin, conventionally all factors affecting dust formation can be divided into mining and geological and industrial-technical. The former determines the amount of dust and rock formed during coal destruction (content of free SiO_2, strength, moisture content and composition of coal substances, etc.), the others determine the transition of dust into a suspended state (method and mode of coal destruction, power and angle of formation dip, air speed, etc.) [28].

Limited reserves of functioning of any system under conditions of extreme regulation are not able to provide sufficient resistance of the organism to the influence of above-normative in terms of intensity and duration of industrial dust parameters for a long time at the expense of compensatory-adaptive mechanisms. To control these processes, the technology of sanitary and hygienic monitoring has been developed [29].

Pneumoconiosis and COPD of occupational etiology have a common etiological factor—industrial pollutants. But the basis of the pathogenesis of pneumoconiosis is the formation of coniotic granulomas in the lung parenchyma, regional lymphatic system, and perivascular, peribronchial, and intermediate fibrosis. The basis of the pathogenesis of COPD of occupational etiology is the lesion of the bronchial mucosa and the formation of diffuse catarrhal, sub- or atrophic endobronchitis, and peribronchitis with further formation of broncho-obstructive syndrome [30].

Many aspects are underdeveloped in DRD: (1) the duration of relatively safe work experience in dusty conditions and the timing of the onset of pathology; (2) determination of the initial signs of pathology development in all lung structures of preclinical and dorentgenological character; (3) clinical variant establishment of dust pathology; (4) the ratio of chronic dust bronchitis and pneumoconiosis, and so on [31, 32].

The objective of the present work was to create a mathematical risk model for the development of pneumoconiosis (Pn) and chronic obstructive pulmonary disease (COPD) based on hygienic, functional, and clinical indicators.

2. Material and methods

The research was conducted on 530 patients during 2011–2019. All the patients were coal miners who were hospitalized in the therapeutic department of the Republican Centre for Occupational Pathology and Rehabilitation (RCPAR) in Donetsk with diagnoses: Pn (Main 1 group, n = 244) and COPD (Main 2 group, n = 286). The comparison group consisted of relatively healthy long-term dust-contacted miners (n = 47), who were selected by random sampling, randomized by age and experience, and whose working conditions coincided with those of the main group. No diseases of internal organs and nervous system were detected in the comparison group. The control group consisted of healthy donors (n = 52). The groups of patients with Pn and COPD under study included coal miners from one city, one district, one mine, one site, and one occupational group (**Table 1**).

Coal seams in Donbass are laid down at different angles of inclination to the horizontal surface and are divided into gentle (from 0 to 18°), inclined (from 19 to 35°), inclined steeply (from 36 to 55°), and steep seams (from 56 to 90°) [33]. Depending on the bedding of the coal seams, the mines studied were divided into mines with steep bedding (Gorlovka, Enakievo) and mines with gentle bedding (Donetsk, Makeevka, Khartsyzsk, Torez). Depending on the degree of direct contact in work with dust, all mining occupations were divided into three groups: (1) mining site (longwall face): stope miner, face miner, operator of rock removing machines, mining foreman, coal combine operator, site manager, site mechanic, underground miner, and mining fitter; (2) mine face: shaft man, timber man, shotfirer, mine worker on repair of mine workings, and drill runner; (3) auxiliary: electric fitter,

Indicator	Groups of studied people			
	Main 1 (n = 244)	Main 2 (n = 286)	Comparison (n = 47)	Control (n = 52)
Cortisol (mol/l)	$288.71 \pm 17.07^{*,\&}$	$421.69 \pm 39.35^{\#}$	456.15 ± 15.23^{x}	369.00 ± 29.86
DC (U/ml)	$3.67 \pm 1.28^{*,\&}$	$2.38 \pm 0.82^{\#}$	3.42 ± 1.03^{x}	1.95 ± 0.44
MD (kmol/gr protein)	$10.23 \pm 2.15^{*,\&}$	$11.68 \pm 2.96^{\#}$	8.40 ± 1.93^{x}	6.11 ± 1.53
PAA (%)	$48.67 \pm 10.33^{*,\&}$	$46.08 \pm 8.25^{\#}$	54.70 ± 10.61	57.10 ± 5.12
Catalase (mkat/l)	$13.57 \pm 5.35^{*,\&}$	$11.78 \pm 5.02^{\#}$	16.38 ± 4.20^{x}	18.13 ± 3.86
Vitamin E (kmol /l)	$3.58 \pm 1.38^{*,\&}$	$4.28 \pm 1.08^{\#}$	4.70 ± 1.27	5.14 ± 0.88
UA (mmol/l)	$0.56 \pm 0.15^{*,\&}$	$0.45 \pm 0.11^{\#}$	0.32 ± 0.13^{x}	0.25 ± 0.07
XO (ncatal/l)	$5.80 \pm 1.39^{*,\&}$	$4.03 \pm 1.08^{\#}$	2.63 ± 0.77^{x}	1.68 ± 0.33

$^{*}p < 0.05$ (t)—Main 1 and Control.$^{\#}p < 0.05$ (t)—Main 2 and Control.$^{x}p < 0.05$ (t)—Comparisons and Control. $^{\&}p < 0.05$ (t)—Main 1 and Main 2.

Table 1.
Differences in immunological and biochemical parameters in four groups: Main 1 (Pn), Main 2 (COPD), Comparisons (dust-exposed miners), Control (healthy donors).

electric locomotive driver, underground tipping machine operator, hoisting machine operator, and operator of rock removing machines.

Dust pollution of workplaces was assessed by the generally accepted method.

The general blood analysis was performed on the cytological analyzer COBAS EMIRA (La ROCHE, Austria) (on the basis of RCPAR) with determination of the number of erythrocytes, hemoglobin, color index, number of leukocytes, lymphocytes, mononuclear cells, neutrophils, and erythrocyte sedimentation rate (ESR) [34].

Spirography is a method of graphic registration of changes in lung volumes during respiratory movements. All indicators of pulmonary ventilation are divided conditionally into static or anatomical—lung volumes—and functional—indicators of pulmonary ventilation directly. These indices are variable, and they depend on sex, age, weight, height, body position, the state of the nervous system, and so on. The indices are recorded in the quiet mode. The indices are recorded in the mode of quiet breathing and some during forced maneuvers [35].

Calculations were performed using the license packages 'Statistica 7' (Start Soft Rus) and 'Stadia 6.1' ('Informatics and Computers', Moscow). To compare the main and control groups, descriptive statistics and nonparametric criterion to assess reliability (Mann-Whitney U test) were used. Since some indicators do not obey the normal distribution law based on the results of such criteria as Kolmogorov-Smirnov Normality test, Shapiro-WilkW-test, kurtosis coefficient, standard error of Kurtosis, Skewness, and standard error of Skewness, the data set was transformed logarithmically ($\log10(x)$) to work further and solve problems. The construction of risk models for the development of pneumoconiosis and chronic obstructive pulmonary disease in miners was performed using general discriminant analysis (GDA).

3. Results

According to the results of spirography, it was found that forced vital capacity of lungs (FVCL) in Pn patients was reduced significantly (2.61 ± 0.75 l) in comparison with control (4.35 ± 0.53 l) ($St = 12.87$, $p < 0.0001$). The situation is similar between FVCL level in COPD patients and FVCL level in controls (2.45 ± 0.60 l and 4.35 ± 0.53 l, respectively) ($St = 15.19$, $p < 0.0001$). Also, FVCL was reduced in the comparison group (3.59 ± 0.54 l) in contrast to control (4.35 ± 0.53 l) ($St = 11.02$, $p < 0.0001$). Differences between other groups by this indicator were statistically unreliable ($St = 0.96$, $p > 0.05$). According to the results of spirography of forced expiratory volume in 1 second (FEV1), it was found that FEV1 in Pn patients was reduced significantly (1.82 ± 0.65) l compared to control (3.57 ± 0.45 l) ($St = 14.94$, $p < 0.0001$). The situation is similar between the level of FEV1 in COPD patients and in controls (1.65 ± 0.57 l and 3.57 ± 0.45 l, respectively) ($St = 17.17$, $p < 0.0001$). Also, this index was reduced in the comparison group (3.05 ± 0.41) l in contrast to control (3.57 ± 0.45) l ($St = 10.51$, $p < 0.0001$). Differences between Pn and COPD on this index are statistically unreliable ($St = 1.18$, $p > 0.05$). According to the results of spirography of the level of peak volumetric forced expiratory flow rate (PVF), it was found that PVF in patients with Pn is reduced significantly (3.95 ± 1.82 l/s) compared to control (8.37 ± 0.81 l/s) ($St = 15.41$, $p < 0.0001$). A similar situation was observed between the level of PVF in COPD patients and that of controls (3.65 ± 1.40 l/s and 8.37 ± 0.81 l/s, respectively) ($St = 19.56$, $p < 0.0001$). Also, this index was slightly reduced in the comparison group (6.18 ± 0.98 l/s) in contrast to the control (8.37 ± 0.81 l/s) (St = 10.12, $p < 0.0001$). Differences between Pn and COPD were unreliable statistically (St = 0.76, $p > 0.05$).

According to the results of cortisol level study, it was found that cortisol in Pn patients was reduced compared to control (St = 4.22, $p < 0.0001$). Similar dynamics are visualized between cortisol level in Pn patients and cortisol level in COPD patients (St = 7.29, $p < 0.0001$). In addition, cortisol in COPD patients is significantly higher than in controls (St = 2.49, $p < 0.05$). The same trend is observed between cortisol levels in the comparison group and cortisol levels in controls (St = 4.19, $p < 0.0001$). According to the results of the study of diene conjugates (DC) level, it was found that DC in Pn patients was increased significantly compared to controls (St = 9.26, $p < 0.0001$). Similar dynamics are noted between the level of DC in COPD patients and the level of DC in controls (St = 3.58, $p < 0.001$), as well as in the comparison of this index in the comparison group and in controls (St = 9.28, $p < 0.0001$). In addition, DC level was higher in Pn patients than in COPD patients (St = 8.91, $p < 0.0001$). According to the results of the study of malonic dialdehyde (MD) level, it was found that MD was elevated in Pn patients compared to controls (St = 11.95, $p < 0.0001$). Similar dynamics are noted between MD level in COPD patients and MD level in control (St = 12.71, $p < 0.0001$), as well as in comparison of this index between comparison group and control (St = 6.52, $p < 0.0001$). In addition, MD was higher in COPD patients than in Pn patients (St = 3.89, $p < 0.001$). According to the results of the study of plasma antioxidant activity (PAA) level, it was found that PAA in Pn patients was significantly reduced compared to control (St = 5.43, $p < 0.0001$). A similar dynamic is visualized between PAA levels in COPD patients and PAA levels in controls (St = 8.85, $p < 0.0001$). In addition, PAA in Pn patients is slightly higher than in COPD patients (St = 2.02, $p < 0.05$). According to the results of the study of catalase (Cat) level, it was found that catalase was significantly reduced in Pn patients compared to controls (St = 5.32, $p < 0.0001$). The situation is similar between the level of Cat in COPD patients and the level of Cat in control (St = 8.09, $p < 0.0001$), as well as in the comparison of this index between the comparison group and control (St = 2.13, $p < 0.05$). In addition, Cat in Pn patients is slightly higher than in COPD patients (St = 2.47, $p < 0.05$). According to the results of vitamin E level study, it was found that vitamin E was significantly decreased in Pn patients compared to control (St = 7.21, $p < 0.0001$). A similar situation is noted between the level of vitamin E in COPD patients and the level of vitamin E in controls (St = 5.03, $p < 0.0001$). In addition to the above in the comparison of this index, the vitamin E level in COPD patients is higher than in Pn patients (St = 4.12, $p < 0.0001$). According to the results of the study of uric acid (UA) level, it was found that UA is significantly increased in Pn patients compared to controls (St = 13.34, $p < 0.0001$). Similar dynamics are noted between the level of UA in COPD patients and UA level in controls (St = 11.06, $p < 0.0001$). Also, this index is slightly increased in the comparison group in contrast to the control (St = 3.15, $p < 0.01$). In addition, UA in Pn patients is significantly higher than in COPD patients (St = 5.78, $p < 0.0001$). According to the results of xanthine oxidase (XO) level, it was found that XO was significantly increased in Pn patients compared to controls (St = 20.77, $p < 0.0001$). A similar situation is observed between the level of XO in COPD patients and the level of XO in controls (St = 15.20, $p < 0.0001$). This index is slightly increased in the comparison group in contrast to the control (St = 8.04, $p < 0.0001$). In addition, the level of XO is significantly higher in Pn patients than in COPD patients (St = 10.42, $p < 0.001$) (**Table 1**).

Factors	Factor value	% of explained cumulative variance	Cumulative value of the factor	Cumulative %
Factor 1	6.899062	21.55957	6.89906	21.55957
Factor 2	3.171990	9.91247	10.07105	31.47204
Factor 3	2.735712	8.54910	12.80676	40.02114

Table 2.
Explained cumulative variance of pneumoconiosis factors on M2 array.

To solve the set tasks, the matrix for patients with the studied diseases (Pn and COPD) was distributed into three arrays in each nosology: Array 1: hygienic indices, spirography indices, general blood analysis; Array 2: hygienic indices, spirography indices, general blood analysis, biochemical blood analysis; Array 3: hygienic indices, spirography indices, general blood analysis, biochemical blood analysis, immunological indices. The classification of the above arrays is based on the principles of simplicity and availability of research methods (from simple to complex and from cheaper to more expensive). Factor analysis was used to determine the structure of the disease under study, as well as the architectonics of the interrelationship of the variables under study (**Table 2**).

As a result of the factor analysis, three factors were identified. Factor 1 included the following spirographic indices: Forced vital capacity of the lungs (FVCL), inspiratory vital capacity (IVC), forced expiratory volume in 1 second (FEV1), mean volumetric velocity between 25% and 75% FVCL (M2575), peak expiratory volume velocity (PEV), instantaneous volume velocity after exhalation of 25% FVCL (IVV25), instantaneous volume velocity after exhalation of 50% FVCL (IVV50), and instantaneous volume velocity after exhalation of 75% FVCL (IVV75). Factor 2 included diene conjugates (DC), malonic dialdehyde (MD), and superoxide dismutase (SOD). And Factor 3 combined hygienic parameters such as occupation, actual dust exposure (DEact), and control dust exposure (CDE) (**Table 3**).

These three factors explained ≈40% of the variance of M2 array pneumoconiosis variables (Factor 1—21.56%, Factor 2—9.91%, and Factor 3—8.55%).

As a result of the factor analysis, two factors were identified. Factor 1 included the following spirographic indices: Forced vital capacity of the lungs (FVCL), inspiratory vital capacity (IVC), forced expiratory volume in 1 second (FEV1), mean volumetric velocity between 25% and 75% FVCL (M2575), instantaneous volume velocity after exhalation of 25% FVCL (IVV25), instantaneous volume velocity after exhalation of 50% FVCL (IVV50), and instantaneous volume velocity after exhalation of 75% FVCL (IVV75). Factor 2 combined the hygiene parameters such as occupation, actual dust exposure (ADact), and control dust exposure (CDA).

These two factors explained 30.04% of the variance of chronic obstructive pulmonary disease variables of the M2 array (Factor 1—21.89% and Factor 2—8.15%) (**Table 3**).

General discriminant analysis (GDA) was used to construct a prediction function for the development of disease (pneumoconiosis or COPD) in miners (**Tables 4** and **5**).

As a result of the general discriminant analysis, a disease prediction function (pneumoconiosis or chronic obstructive pulmonary disease) was derived. The predictors of this model are the following variables: Mine type ($p = 0.000336$), forced vital capacity of the lungs (FVC) ($p = 0.001595$), inspiratory vital capacity (IVC)

Factors	Factor value	% of explained cumulative variance	Cumulative value of the factor	Cumulative %
Factor 1	7.007859	21.89956	7.007859	21.89956
Factor 2	2.608115	8.15036	9.615974	30.04992

Table 3.
Explained cumulative variance of COPD factors on the M2 array.

Diseases	Effectiveness	Pn	COPD	Total number in the group
		p = 0.4708	**p = 0.5292**	
Pneumoconiosis (Pn)	88.52459	108.0000	14.0000	122.0000
COPD	94.11765	8.0000	128.0000	136.0000
Total percentage of the model	**91.32112**	116.0000	142.0000	

Table 4.
Function construction on the combined M2 array (combined M2 of pneumoconiosis patients and M2 of COPD patients). Classification matrix of the analyzed sample.

Diseases	Effectiveness	Pn	COPD	Total number in the group
		p = 0.4708	**p = 0.5292**	
Pneumoconiosis (Pn)	73.13432	49.0000	12.0000	61.0000
COPD	91.17647	6.0000	62.0000	68.0000
Total percentage of the model	**82.15539**	55.0000	78.0000	

Table 5.
Cross-validation classification matrix.

($p = 0.000240$), cortisol ($p = 0.000004$), diene conjugates ($p = 0.000001$), malonic dialdehyde ($p = 0.000002$), antioxidant activity plasma ($p = 0.006769$), catalase ($p = 0.000302$), vitamin E ($p = 0.000001$), uric acid ($p = 0.000376$), and xanthine oxidase ($p = 0.000002$).

Taking into account the coefficients assigned to the mentioned variables, the function has the following form:

$$\begin{aligned}\text{Pn} = -347.565 + 40.224^{*}\ \text{FVCL} - 25.235^{*}\ \text{IVC} + 73.876^{*}\ \text{Cortisol} + 20.640^{*}\ \text{DC}\\ +110.501^{*}\ \text{MD} + 232.237^{*}\ \text{PAA} - 26.642^{*}\ \text{Catalase} - 7.574^{*}\ \text{Vit.}E - 29.078^{*}\ \text{UA}\\ +30.400^{*}\ \text{XO} + 1.036^{*}\ \text{Shafts (type1)}.\end{aligned} \quad (1)$$

$$\begin{aligned}\text{COPD} = -359.417 + 27.205^{*}\ \text{FVCL} - 9.868^{*}\ \text{IVC} + 79.843^{*}\ \text{Cortisol} + 8.849^{*}\ \text{DC}\\ +128.693^{*}\ \text{MD} + 224.428^{*}\ \text{PAA} - 32.117^{*}\ \text{Catalase} + 2.212^{*}\ \text{Vit.}E - 35.974^{*}\ \text{UA}\\ +21.894^{*}\ \text{XO} + 1.930^{*}\ \text{Shafts (type1)}.\end{aligned} \quad (2)$$

Based on the classification matrix of the analyzed sample (2/3rd of the total sample size in proportion to each disease), the effectiveness of the model in predicting the development of the diseases under study is 91.32% (pneumoconiosis—88.52% and COPD—94.11%). Model correctness is 82.15% (pneumoconiosis and COPD—73.13% and 91.17%, respectively) with cross-validation (1/3rd of the total sample size in proportion to each disease).

When working with Array 2, three factors were identified as a result of factor analysis for pneumoconiosis patients. Factor 1 included the following spirographic indices: FVCL, IVC, FEV1, M2575, PVF, IVV 25, IVV 50, IVV 75. Factor 2 included: DC, MD, and SOD. And Factor 3 combined hygiene parameters such as: occupation, DEact, and CDE. These three factors explain $\approx$ 40% of the variance of variables Pn of Array 2. When working with Array 2, two factors were identified as a result of the factor analysis performed on COPD patients. Factor 1 included the following spirographic indices: FVCL, IVC, FEV1, M2575, IVV25, IVV50, and IVV75. Factor 2 combined such hygienic parameters as: occupation, DEact, and CDE. These two factors explained 30.04% of the variance of COPD variables of Array 2.

The technology of sanitary and hygienic monitoring of working conditions based on the assessment of occupational route, seniority dose of harmful factor, and individual occupational risks was developed for coal miners. Occupational routes of coal mine workers were studied, their main types were determined, and occupational risks were calculated.

The underground method of coal mining has a number of specific characteristics. According to the results of the assessment of workers' professional routes for underground operations in a typical coal mine, it was found that only some miners' professions are strictly 'tied' to the production site, workplace, and type of activity: drill runners, hoist drivers, electric locomotive operators, powder men, and shotfirers. The following are not 'tied': mine workers at the mine face—are part of the staff of the mining, tunneling, equipment installation, dismantling, and adjustment sections; operator of rock removing machines—part of the mining, tunneling, and capital mining sections; tunnellers and mine fitters—part of the mining, tunneling, capital mining sections and installation, dismantling, and setting up of equipment; mine workmen for repair of mine workings and mine workers of underground installations are employed in more than half of mine production areas; and underground mine workers, underground electricians, and mine foremen—at practically all production sites.

Among miners in the main occupations, less than 10% of workers do not change their occupation, 44% of workers change their profession once, 30%—twice, and the remaining 17%—three or more times. Almost half of auxiliary miners do not change their occupation. One-third change their occupation once, and 20–25%—two or more times.

Thus, throughout the whole labor experience of a coal mining worker, there is a constant change of working conditions at underground workplaces. For many decades, hygienic assessment of labor conditions provided for the use of the existing normative base, which is presented in the form of MPC and MPL of harmful production factors. To control working conditions, the state services for hygiene and labor protection previously had approved procedures for attestation of workplaces, which was carried out routinely at least once every 5 years.

In this form, the control system does not provide personalized information on workers' working conditions and health status. Actual data on these issues are presented in the form of impersonal units of cases of non-compliance of labor conditions with hygienic standards, cases of first detected occupational or production-related diseases, and so on. Such information cannot be sufficient to reveal the mechanisms of development of pathological processes in the organism, to predict the terms of occupational health violation, to establish the degree of negative impact of working conditions on workers, to identify the cause-and-effect relationship of diseases with specific working conditions, to justify individual measures to prevent diseases, and so on. In this case, the main meaning and purpose of hygienic analysis is lost.

To assess the accumulated impact of labor conditions on workers over time, the occupational itinerary is studied in the form of a time-ordered chain (list) of enterprises, production sites, workshops, services, and professions (specialties, positions), where a person has worked during his/her working life, taking into account the period of work at each workplace. The status of an occupational route is legally secured by entries in the employment history. Hygienic assessment of an occupational route is the study of sanitary and hygienic parameters of labor conditions for compliance of workplaces (which constitute an occupational route) with current hygienic standards, sanitary rules and norms, with determination of the accumulated (seniority) (over-normative) dose of exposure to harmful production factors, and with the corresponding occupational risk of health impairment. The last type of research is especially important for industries, where a majority of production factors have chronic impact exclusively or predominantly, and the biological effect of more than 90% of this is registered in the form of chronic occupational pathology.

Control of exposure of workers to industrial dust provides for accounting:

- the degree to which the actual dust concentration exceeds the maximum permissible value;
- pulmonary ventilation during work;
- work experience in conditions of dust exposure (dust length of service).

Passport data, data on air dustiness in the workplace, and the employee's occupational route and labor activity are filled in **Table 6**.

Table 7 is prepared on the basis of the data in **Table 6**. The algorithm for calculating the average values of the degree of dust exceeding the MPC and pulmonary ventilation for the whole period of work in conditions of industrial dust exposure provides summarizing the number of worked shifts, separately for each multiplicity of dust exceeding the MPC and at each level of pulmonary ventilation with the subsequent determination of the fractional value and the average time-weighted value by summing up the fractional values.

The risk was calculated depending on the multiplicity of dust concentration exceedance relative to the standard (an example of 1.1–2.0 times exceedance of MPC; **Table 8**).

Personal data in a systematized form on the impact of working conditions on miners' health can be used to develop and implement therapeutic and diagnostic, therapeutic and preventive, and rehabilitation measures during preliminary and periodic medical examinations, professional selection, employment, granting benefits for work in harmful conditions, workers' health improvement, and check-ups. Implementation of the study results in practice will lead to a decrease in the level of occupationally caused and occupational morbidity, increase in the period of work in harmful and hazardous conditions before occupational disease development, and

Full name	Employee number	Identification number 1	Enterprise	Production site. Service	Occupation (position)	Workplace	Date of work			Technology characteristics	Equipment characteristics	Source of dust formation	Average daily dust concentration, mg/m^3	Dust MPC. $мг/м^3$	Multiplicity of MPC exceedance	Average daily lung ventilation, m^3/min
							beginning	end	Calender days							
1	2	3	4	5	6	7	8	9	10	11	12	13	14	15	16	17

Table 6.
Data on analyzing the impact of industrial dust on the worker.

Full name	MPC Dust Exposure Ratio	Average lung ventilation m^3/min.	Calendar days sum	Sum* working shifts	Average value of dust exceedance multiplicity relative to MPC	Mean pulmonary ventilation
	(C_i/ MPC_i)	(Q_i)	(n_i)	(z_i)	($D_i = C_i/MPC_i \times z_i/\sum z_i$)	($D_i = Q_i \times z_i/\sum z_i$)
IonovR.S.	5	0.029	256	154	1.59	0.0092
	7	0.030	153	92	1.33	0.0057
	4	0.032	36	22	0.18	0.0014
	3	0.028	136	82	0.51	0.0047
	5	0.033	225	135	1.39	0.0092
				$\sum z_i = 485$	$\sum D_i = 5.0$	$\sum D_i = 0.0302$

To calculate the number of working shifts, the sum of calendar days is multiplied by the coefficient 0.6027.

Table 7.
Algorithm to calculate the multiplicity of dust exceeding MPC and pulmonary ventilation on average during the period of work when exposed to industrial dust.

increase in the effectiveness of prevention of health disorders, including occupational diseases and their complications (disability), and of patients' rehabilitation.

4. Discussion

The prediction model for pneumoconiosis in coal workers using machine learning algorithms was established in Dong et al. [36]. Clinical data were with significant differences including arterial blood gas analysis, lung function test, blood cell analysis, inflammatory markers, blood biochemical parameters, coagulation function, and serum oncomarkers. This dataset consisted of 62 clinical parameters collected, all of which were continuous variables. The data obtained by the authors are consistent with our data but reflect the prediction of only one disease, namely pneumoconiosis [36].China is one of the countries with the highest incidence of occupational pneumoconiosis in the world [7–9]. It accounted for 85–90% of all annually reported occupational diseases in China over the past decade [10]. According to the Chinese Pneumoconiosis Diagnostic Standard, diagnoses are made based on occupational history, physical examination, chest radiographs, and pulmonary function tests (National Health and Family Planning Commission of the People's Republic of China, 2014). In this study, epidemiological data from 1963 to 2014 on nearly 9000 Chinese miners were analyzed to predict trends in CWP incidence. GARCH and ARIMA time series models were used. GARCH more accurately modeled the historical variability of CWP rates over time compared to ARIMA. Although overall incidence decreased with dustiness reduction, risk levels remained elevated. Both models failed to predict accurately short-term trends, emphasizing the importance of ongoing occupational surveillance combined with improved exposure tracking to better protect workers from preventable respiratory disease [37].

Compared with controls, the distinctive biomarkers of CWP were severe alveolitis, severe goblet cell hyperplasia (GCH), severe hyperplastic epithelial changes, and severe squamous metaplasia. Multivariate analysis showed that severe alveolitis and severe GCH, along with the miner's duration of employment and current smoking,

Work experience years	Occupational risk (%) at pulmonary ventilation volume (m^3/min)												
	0.016	0.018	0.02	0.022	0.024	0.026	0.028	0.03	0.032	0.034	0.036	0.38	0.04
1	2	3	4	5	6	7	8	9	10	11	12	13	14
5	2.5	2.7	3.0	3.2	3.5	3.7	3.9	4.2	4.4	4.7	4.9	5.1	5.4
6	3.0	3.3	3.6	3.9	4.2	4.5	4.7	5.0	5.3	5.6	5.9	6.2	6.5
7	3.5	3.8	4.1	4.5	4.8	5.1	5.4	5.8	6.1	6.4	6.7	7.1	7.4
8	4.1	4.4	4.8	5.2	5.6	6.0	6.4	6.8	7.2	7.6	7.9	8.3	8.7
9	4.5	5.0	5.4	5.9	6.3	6.7	7.2	7.6	8.0	8.5	8.9	9.4	9.8
10	5.1	5.6	6.0	6.5	7.0	7.5	8.0	8.5	8.9	9.4	9.9	10.4	10.9
11	5.5	6.0	6.6	7.1	7.7	8.2	8.7	9.3	9.8	10.3	10.9	11.4	12.0
12	6.0	6.6	7.2	7.8	8.4	9.0	9.5	10.1	10.7	11.3	11.9	12.5	13.0
13	6.6	7.2	7.8	8.5	9.1	9.7	10.3	11.0	11.6	12.2	12.9	13.5	14.1
14	7.0	7.7	8.4	9.1	9.8	10.4	11.1	11.8	12.5	13.2	13.8	14.5	15.2
15	7.6	8.3	9.0	9.7	10.4	11.2	11.9	12.6	13.3	14.1	14.8	15.5	16.2
16	8.0	8.8	9.6	10.4	11.1	11.9	12.7	13.4	14.2	15.0	15.7	16.5	17.3
17	8.6	9.4	10.2	11.0	11.8	12.6	13.5	14.3	15.1	15.9	16.7	17.5	18.4
18	9.1	9.9	10.8	11.7	12.5	13.4	14.2	15.1	16.0	16.8	17.7	18.6	19.4
19	9.6	10.5	11.4	12.3	13.3	14.2	15.1	16.0	16.9	17.8	18.7	19.6	20.6
20	10.1	11.1	12.0	13.0	13.9	14.9	15.9	16.8	17.8	18.7	19.7	20.6	21.6
21	10.6	11.6	12.6	13.7	14.7	15.7	16.7	17.7	18.7	19.7	20.7	21.8	22.8
22	11.1	12.1	13.2	14.2	15.3	16.3	17.4	18.4	19.5	20.5	21.6	22.6	23.7
23	11.7	12.8	13.9	15.0	16.1	17.3	18.4	19.5	20.6	21.7	22.8	24.0	25.1
24	12.1	13.3	14.5	15.6	16.8	18.0	19.1	20.3	21.5	22.6	23.8	25.0	26.1
25	12.7	13.9	15.1	16.3	17.5	18.7	19.9	21.1	22.3	23.5	24.8	26.0	27.2
26	13.1	14.4	15.6	16.9	18.2	19.4	20.7	21.9	23.2	24.4	25.7	27.0	28.2
27	13.7	15.0	16.3	17.6	18.9	20.2	21.5	22.8	24.1	25.4	26.7	28.0	29.3
28	14.1	15.5	16.9	18.2	19.6	20.9	22.3	23.6	25.0	26.3	27.7	29.0	30.4
29	14.7	16.1	17.5	18.9	20.3	21.7	23.1	24.5	25.9	27.3	28.7	30.1	31.5
30	15.2	16.6	18.1	19.5	21.0	22.4	23.8	25.3	26.7	28.2	29.6	31.1	32.5

Table 8.
Occupational risk from exposure to industrial dust exceeding MPC by 1.1–2.0 times.

were independent predictors of pulmonary mortality. Survival analysis revealed significant differences in survival between the three groups: no evidence of severe alveolitis and severe GCH, presence of severe alveolitis or severe GCH but not both, and both severe alveolitis and severe GCH. Conclusions: The severities of alveolitis and goblet cell hyperplasia on bronchoscopic examination are independent prognostic factors for CWP. A pathology classification system based on these two parameters can be used in the stratification and clinical management of patients with CWP [38].

Comprehensive preventive measures to control nonorganic retroperitoneal tumors, which are currently being implemented in China's state mines, are cost-effective. Engineering control with integrated measures is considered to be more cost-effective than personal protective equipment. Investment in engineering controls should be increased to improve the cost-effectiveness of nonorganic retroperitoneal tumor prevention [21].

Statistically significant differences between biochemical (increased concentration of ceruloplasmin and α-1-antitrypsin) and immunological parameters (increased total number of leukocytes, and ESR, increased concentration of IgG) in miners with chronic dust bronchitis and coal industry workers without this pathology were revealed. The dependence of functional changes in the respiratory system with the development of occupational pathology was determined. Statistically significant decrease of functional indices (volume of forced expiratory volume per second and vital capacity of lungs) and strengthening of degree of respiratory insufficiency were revealed in the persons of the main group. The predisposition to the development of dust bronchitis in holders of HP 1-1 genotype and resistance to the formation of this pathology in persons with HP 2-2 genotype were found. When studying the deletion polymorphism of GSTT 1, it was revealed that carriers of GSTT 1 "+" variant are most susceptible to the development of chronic dust bronchitis, and the owners of GSTT 1 "–" variant were resistant to its formation. A positive association with the development of dust bronchitis in the owners of MM phenotype (MN system) was revealed [39].

1. In patients with non-alcoholic steatohepatitis, NASH on the background of COPD of dust etiology clearly expressed signs of lipoperoxidation activation characterized by an increase in serum concentration of intermediate (DC) and final (MD) lipid peroxidation products, and an increase in erythrocyte peroxidative hemolysis index was revealed. This indicated the negative influence of COPD of dust etiology on pathogenetic mechanisms. Hepatic stenosis was formed in terms of increased processes of lipid layer peroxidation of hepatocyte biomembranes.

2. At application of conventional therapy in the examined patients, there was a decrease in the content of intermediate (DC) and final (MD) lipoperoxidation products and erythrocyte peroxidative hemolysis index in the blood serum, but complete normalization of the studied parameters did not occur.

3. Based on the obtained data, it may be appropriate to analyze the possible effectiveness of the use of drugs with antioxidant properties in patients with NASH on the background of COPD of dust etiology [40].

4. 6-minute walking test (6MWT) evaluation in workers of dust hazardous occupations should be carried out taking into account the ventilation function, diffusion capacity, echoCG results, and the level of power developed during the test.

5. Tolerance to physical load in dust workers is determined by airway patency, the severity of emphysema, fibrotic changes, and myocardial contractility, left and right heart involvement.

6. Correlation of saturation on the background of physical load with respiratory function indices can be a diagnostic criterion of early manifestations of various variants of dust pathology development [41].

The main changes in miners' bronchi include a sharp decrease in the thickness of the epithelial layer and the severity of its folding; development of sclerosis in the bronchial wall in the form of thickening of the basal membrane and thickening of the intrinsic lamina of the bronchial wall, bronchial glands, and smooth muscle cells hypertrophy, as well as in the development of muff-like peribronchial sclerosis. These processes developed diffusely throughout the whole bronchial tree and by the character of changes corresponded to the concept of primary atrophic bronchopathy.

Histologically, the bronchi showed thinning and disturbance of the epithelial layer architectonics with uneven 'atypical' cell arrangement, loosening and sloughing of cells, decrease in the number of goblet cells, focal proliferation of basal cells and their focal metaplasia into multilayer squamous epithelium, cystic 'rebirth' of bronchial glands, local mononuclear infiltration and muscular layer atrophy, bronchial lumen deformation, and peribronchial sclerosis [42].

The obtained mathematical models of predicting and early diagnosis of pneumoconiosis in galvanic production workers besides the effects on the human body of dust and aerosol fibrogenic risk factors take into account unfavorable environmental factors of other nature in combination with the ergonomical peculiarities of galvanic shops and with individual risk factors. The obtained model with the use of methods of expert evaluations and mathematical modeling was shown to provide confidence in the correct prediction of occurrence and development of pneumoconiosis of galvanic production workers not lower than 0.85 and early diagnosis not lower than 0.9 [43].

5. Conclusion

The mathematical model of pneumoconiosis and chronic obstructive pulmonary disease development risk has been created (efficiency 91.32%, correctness 82.15%) on the basis of hygienic, functional, and clinical indicators.

Author details

Olga Yurievna Nikolenko*, Dmitry Olegovich Lastkov, Oleg Viktorovich Partas and Inna Sergeevna Eromyants
Federal State Budgetary Educational Institution of Higher Education "M. Gorky Donetsk State Medical University" of the Ministry of Health of the Russian Federation, Donetsk, Russian Federation

*Address all correspondence to: olegpartas@mail.ru

References

[1] Onishhenko GG. Professional'naya zabolevaemost' v sovremenny'x social'no-e'konomicheskix usloviyax Donbassa [Tekst]. Medicinatrudaipromy' shlennayae'kologiya. 2022;**62**(10): 630-639

[2] Novikova EA. Povyshenie bezopasnosti konveyernogo transporta v gornakh vyrabotkakh ugol'nykh shakht: monografiya. Dnepropetrovsk: Natsional'nyy gornyy universitet; 2013. 99 p

[3] Kryuchkova EN, Saarkoppel' LM, Yatsyna IV. Osobennosti immunnogo otveta pri khronicheskom vozdeystvii promyshlennykh aerozoley. Gigiena i Sanitariya. 2016;**95**(11):1058-1061

[4] Zemskov AN, Liskova MY, Smirnova EV. Analiz usloviy truda gornorabochikh i meropriyatiya po normalizatsii pylevogo i gazovogo sostava atmosfery shakht i rudnikov. Izvestie TulGU. Nauki o Zemle. 2017;**2**: 58-68

[5] Babanov SA, Budash DS. Dokazatel'nost', professional'nye riski i biologicheskie markery pri professional'nykh zabolevaniyakh legkikh. Meditsina truda i ekologiya cheloveka. 2018;**1**:34-43

[6] Vanka KS, Shukla S, Gomez HM, James C, Palanisami T, Williams K, et al. Understanding the pathogenesis of occupational coal and silica dust-associated lung disease. European Respiratory Review. 2022;**31**(165): 210250. DOI: 10.1183/ 16000617.0250-2021. Print 2022 Sep 30.

[7] Donaldson K, Wallace WA, MacNee W, Henry C, Seaton A. The recognition of lung disease in coal workers: The role of Gough-Wentworth whole lung sections. The Journal of the Royal College of Physicians of Edinburgh. 2022;**52**(1):65-72. DOI: 10.1177/14782715221088982

[8] He W, Jin N, Deng H, Zhao Q, Yuan F, Chen F, et al. Workers' occupational dust exposure and pulmonary function assessment: Cross-sectional study in China. International Journal of Environmental Research and Public Health. 2022;**19**(17):11065. DOI: 10.3390/ijerph191711065

[9] Kurenkova GV, Lemeshevskaya EP. Gigienicheskaya kharakteristika usloviy truda v podzemnykh sooruzheniyakh i ikh vliyanie na zdorov'e rabotnikov. Sibirskiy Meditsinskiy Zhurnal (Irkutsk). 2015;**5**:98-105

[10] Sukhova AV, Gvozdeva LL, Lutsenko LA. O sovershenstvovanii kriteriev otsenki pylevoy nagruzki dlya zashchity zdorov'ya rabotnikov pylevykh professiy V sbornike: aktual'nye voprosy analiza riska pri obespechenii sanitarno-epidemiologicheskogo blagopoluchiya naseleniya i zashchity prav potrebiteley. In: Materialy IX Vserossiyskoy nauchno-prakticheskoy konferentsii s Permskii natsional'nyi issledovatel'skii politekhnicheskii universitet, Perm'. 2019. pp. 704-711

[11] Fomenko DV, Ulanova EV, Zoloeva PV. [i dr.] Kliniko-eksperimental'noe issledovanie metabolicheskikh izmeneniy organizma pri dlitel'no vdykhanii ugol'no-porodnoy pyli. Byulleten' SO RAMN. 2010;**30**(1): 117-122

[12] McGuire C. Dust to Dust. Lancet Respiratory Medicine. 2019;**7**(5):

383-384. DOI: 10.1016/S2213-2600(19)30116-X. Epub 2019 Apr 5

[13] Timofeeva SS, Murzin MA. Pylevaya nagruzka pri dobyche uglya i professional'nye riski. Vestnik IrGTU. 2015;**100**(5):68-71

[14] Katola VM, Komogortseva VE. Pyl': istochniki obrazovaniya, ee obshchaya kharakteristika, pylevye zabolevaniya (kratkiy obzor). Byulleten'. 2018;**67**: 111-116

[15] Sharov NA, Dudaev RR, Krishchuk DI, Liskova MY. Metody pylepodavleniya na ugol'nykh razrezakh Kraynego Severa. Vestnik PNIPU. Geologiya. Neftegazovoe i gornoe delo. 2019;**19**(2):184-200

[16] Davydov SYa, Valiev NG, Suslov NM, Semin AN, Ermolaeva AI, Cheremisina TN, Filatov MS. Pyleobrazovanie i ispol'zovanie pyli gornykh porod na promyshlennykh ob"ektakh. Izvestiya Ural'skogo gosudarstvennogo gornogo univerchsiteta. 2016:**43**(3);87-90

[17] Kislitsyna VV, Motuz IY. Pylevoy faktor na predpriyatiyakh ugol'noy promyshlennosti. Sovremennye nauchnye issledovaniya i innovatsii. 2014;(4). Ch. 2 [Elektronnyy resurs]. Available from: http://web.snauka.ru/issues/2014/04/32001 [Obrashcheniya: 26.03.2019]

[18] Egorova AM, Lutsenko LA, Fedorovich GV, Sukhova AV. Sovershenstvovanie gigienicheskikh kriteriev otsenki hiska zdorov'yu rabotnikov pylevykh professiy. Mezhdunarodnyy zhurnal prikladnykh i fundamental'nykh issledovaniy. 2020; **10**:33-37

[19] Cohen RA, Patel A, Green FH. Lung disease caused by exposure to coal mine and silica dust. Seminars in Respiratory and Critical Care Medicine. 2008;**29**(6): 651-661

[20] Onder M, Onder S. Evaluation of occupational exposures to respirable dust in underground coal mines. Industrial health. 2009;**47**(1):43-49

[21] Ge X, Cui K, Ma H, Zhao S, Meng W, Wang W. Cost-effectiveness of comprehensive preventive measures for coal workers' pneumoconiosis in China. BMC Health Services Research. 2022; **22**(1):266. DOI: 10.1186/s12913-022-07654-7

[22] Perederiya GS, Lastkova DO, Partasa OV. Udoskonalennya sanitarno-gigienichnogo monitoringu vplivu umov pratsi na zdorov'ya girnikiv vugil'nikh shakht: monografiya/Za red. Donets'k: Svit knigi. 2012. 319 p

[23] Zakharenkov VV, Kislitsyna VV. Gigienicheskaya otsenka usloviy truda i professional'nogo riska dlya zdorov'ya rabotnikov ugol'noy shakhty. Uspekhi Sovremennogo Estestvoznaniya. 2013;**11**: 14-18

[24] Zakharenkov VV, Surzhikov DV, Oleshchenko AM, Kislitsyna VV, Korsakova TG, Bol'shakov VV, et al. Klassifikatsiya usloviy truda rabotnikov ugol'nykh razrezov po faktoram riska. Mezhdunarodnyy zhurnal prikladnykh i fundamental'nykh issledovaniy. 2013;**12**: 85-87

[25] Gareeva LF, Gallyamova SA, Masyagutova LM, Akhmetshina VT, Valeeva ET. Clinical and radiological characteristics of pneumoconioses in current conditions. Occupational Health and Human Ecology. 2023;**1**: 35-48

[26] Khalimov YS, Tsepkova GA, Vlasenko AN, Shilov VV,

Andreenko ON. Pozdniy silikoz – redkaya forma pnevmokonioza. Vestnik Rossiyskoy Voenno-meditsinskoy Akademii. 2020;**2**(70):74-78

[27] Izmerov NF, Denisov EI, Molodkina NN, Rodionova GK. Methodology of occupational risk assessment in occupational medicine. Occupational Medicine and Industrial Ecology. 2000;(12):1-7

[28] Chebotarev AG, Gibadulina IY. Kharakteristika rudnichnogo aerozolya i professinal'naya legochnaya patologiya u rabochikh vysokomekhanizirovannykh shakht. Meditsina Truda i Promyshlennaya Ekologiya. 2009;7:7-12

[29] Umans'kiy VY, Perederiy GS, Lastkov DO, ta in. Udoskonalennya kontrolyu za bezpekoyu robit i zdorov'yam shakhtariv na bazi avtomatizovanoї sistemi kompleksnoї bezpeki. Aktual'ni pitannya diagnostiki ta likuvannya profesiynikh zakhvoryuvan' v Ukraïni. Kriviy rig. 2010:72-79

[30] Rubtsov RV. Rol' kliniko-funktsional'nikh doslidzhen' pri pnevmokoniozi v poєdnanni z khronichnim obstruktivnim zakhvoryuvannyam legen' u pratsivnikiv girnichorudnoї ta metalurgiynoї promislovosti. Medichni Perspektivi. 2018;**3**(23):176-181

[31] Bondarev OI, Rykova OV, Razumov VV, Cherdantsev MV, Bugaeva MS. Gistologicheskaya i tsitologicheskaya kharakteristika atroficheskoy bronkhopatii u shakhterov. Meditsina v Kuzbasse. 2012;**4**(1):35-42

[32] Khalimov YS, Tsepkova GA, Vlasenko AN, Shilov VV, Andreenko ON. Late silicosis is a rare form of pneumoconiosis. Bulletin of the Russian Military Medical Academy. 2020;**2**(70):74-78

[33] Mukhin VV. (red.) Meditsina truda v ugol'noy promyshlennosti: Monografiya. Donetsk; 2000. p. 204

[34] Karpishchenko AI. (red.) Meditsinskie laboratornye tekhnologii: Spravochnik. Sankt-Peterburg; 2002. p. 600

[35] Mostoviy YM, Konstantinovich-Chichirel'o TV, Koloshko OM, Rasputina LV. Instrumental'ni metodi doslidzhennya funktsiї zovnishn'ogo dikhannya pri zakhvoryuvannyakh bronkholegenevoї sistemi. Metod. rekomendatsiї. Vinnitsya. 2000:36

[36] Dong H, Zhu B, Kong X, Zhang X. Efficient clinical data analysis for prediction of coal workers' pneumoconiosis using machine learning algorithms. The Clinical Respiratory Journal. 2023;**17**(7):684-693. DOI: 10.1111/crj.13657. Epub 2023 Jun 28

[37] Sun P, Wang B, Zhang H, Xu M, Han L, Zhu B. Medicine (Baltimore). 2024;**103**(7):e37237. DOI: 10.1097/MD.0000000000037237

[38] Cho U, Kim TE, Park CK, Yoon HK, Sa YJ, Kim HL, et al. Prognostic implication of exfoliative airway pathology in cancer-free coal workers' Pneumoconiosis. International Journal of Environmental Research and Public Health. 2022;**19**(22):14975. DOI: 10.3390/ijerph192214975

[39] Kazitskaya AS, Panev NI, Yadykina TK, Gulyaeva ON, Evseeva NA. Geneticheskie i biokhimicheskie aspekty formirovaniya professional'nogo khronicheskogo pylevogo bronkhita Meditsina truda i promyshlennaya ekologiya. 2019;**59**(6):342-347

[40] Miakotkina GV, Sotskaya YaA. Pokazateli lipoperoksidatsii u bol'nykh nealkogol'nym steatogepatitom na fone khronicheskoy obstruktivnoy bolezni legkikh pylevoy etiologii V sbornike: Innovatika v sovremennom mire: opyt, problemy i perspektivy razvitiya. Sbornik nauchnykh statey po materialam XIV Mezhdunarodnoy nauchno-20 fevralya 2024 g., g. Ufa) / - Ufa: Izd. NITS Vestnik nauki. 2024. 137 p

[41] Nenenko OI, Serebryakov PV, Denisova EA. Nagruzochnye proby v diagnostike pylevoy patologii organov dykhaniya Zdravookhranenie Rossiyskoy Federatsii. 2021;**65**(4):384-387

[42] Bondarev OI. Atroficheskie izmeneniya bronkhial'nogo epiteliya kak ranniy skriningovyy marker pylevoy patologii u shakhterov Simvol nauki: mezhdunarodnyy nauchnyy zhurnal. 2023;**3**(1):102-110

[43] Grigorov IY, Khripina II, Serebrovskiy VV, Degtyarev SV. Matematicheskie modeli prognozirovaniya i ranney diagnostiki pnevmokoniozov u rabotnikov gal'vanicheskikh tsekhov. Izvestiya Yugo-Zapadnogo gosudarstvennogo universiteta. Seriya: Upravlenie, vychislitel'naya tekhnika, informatika. Meditsinskoe priborostroenie. 2019;**9**(3):84-98

Chapter 8

Human Factors and Prevention of Medical Errors

Mahdi Jalali

Abstract

Medical errors are a significant concern in healthcare systems, often resulting from complex human factors. This chapter explores the role of human factors in the occurrence of medical errors, with an emphasis on occupational safety and health perspectives that are pertinent to healthcare professionals. By analyzing cognitive, physical, and environmental interactions, we can better understand how these factors lead to errors in healthcare settings. Key frameworks, including the Swiss Cheese Model, Human Factors Analysis and Classification System (HFACS), and the Systems Engineering Initiative for Patient Safety (SEIPS), are evaluated for their utility in mitigating these risks. This chapter provides updated insights and practical recommendations for improving safety in healthcare through enhanced communication, standardized procedures, and targeted training initiatives. The findings underscore the critical need for integrating human factors into healthcare systems to enhance safety and reduce preventable harm, particularly from an occupational health perspective.

Keywords: medical errors, human factors, ergonomics, prevention, healthcare system

1. Introduction

The healthcare system (HCS) is a fundamental aspect of society, consisting of various sectors that promote public health and well-being. Hospitals serve as pivotal components of the HCS, tasked with delivering safe and effective care. However, these facilities can unintentionally become sources of harm due to medical errors. Despite the advancements in medical technology and practices, such errors result in serious complications and fatalities, imposing significant financial burdens on both patients and the healthcare system. Globally, the issue of patient safety has become increasingly pressing, particularly in light of the potential cost savings associated with enhanced safety measures and reduced errors. This focus on safety is in line with occupational safety and health objectives, which aim to create safe working environments for healthcare professionals, whose well-being is directly linked to patient safety [1, 2].

As defined by the Joint Commission on Accreditation of Healthcare Organizations (JCAHO), a medical error is an unintended action caused by negligence that results in an adverse outcome within medical processes. Essentially, a medical error is any action or decision that fails to align with the established HCS standards. These standards are designed to represent well-reasoned and systematic decisions made by authorities based on relevant conditions and requirements. A medical error can either lead to an adverse event or not. An adverse event is defined by three criteria: (1) It must be unfavorable, unwanted, unexpected, and unpredictable; (2) it must involve the participation of healthcare professionals, including doctors and nurses, as well as the hospital or healthcare system; and (3) it should result in actual or potential harm to patients, their families, or the healthcare system as a whole. Adverse events can be either preventable or unavoidable [3].

Given the profound impact of medical errors, there is a growing recognition of the need to focus on human factors in healthcare. This chapter will delve into various human factor considerations—ranging from cognitive errors to systemic issues—and explore practical strategies to prevent medical errors through better design, training, and organizational culture.

1.1 The scope of medical errors in healthcare

According to the definition, a medical error is an unintentional act that arises from negligence and leads to negative consequences during medical procedures. Essentially, it is an action or decision that fails to align with the standards set by the HCS [4, 5].

Errors can occur at any point during the care process: from diagnosis to treatment, follow-up, and even patient communication. These mistakes not only impact patient health outcomes but also contribute to a loss of trust in healthcare systems, leading to an urgent need to focus on prevention.

Previous research indicates that around 10% of patients experience at least one adverse event [6]. Lower-income countries tend to report higher incidences of such events [7]. Recent conservative estimates have positioned patient injury as the 14th leading cause of death worldwide. The World Health Organization (WHO) estimates that there are approximately 421 million hospitalizations globally each year, with about 42.7 million adverse events occurring during these stays [8]. Research shows that, on average, 1 in 10 patients in high-income countries faces an adverse event while receiving hospital care [9]. In low- and middle-income nations, it is estimated that one in four patients suffers harm, leading to roughly 134 million adverse events and approximately 2.6 million deaths annually due to unsafe hospital practices. The global financial impact of medication errors is estimated at $42 billion each year, representing about 1% of total healthcare expenditures [8]. Recent forecasts have suggested that the societal cost of patient harm ranges between $1 trillion and $2 trillion annually. From a human capital perspective, eliminating harm could potentially enhance global economic growth by over 0.7% each year [10]. As a result, prioritizing patient safety and preventing MEs and MAEs in healthcare settings have become an urgent global concern.

1.2 Defining human factors in healthcare

A human factor, also known as ergonomics, is the scientific discipline that examines human interaction with elements of a system. In healthcare, human factors involve understanding how healthcare workers interact with their environment, equipment, technology, and other team members, with the goal of optimizing performance and minimizing errors. The discipline considers a range of elements, including cognitive load, workflow design, communication strategies, and workplace culture [11].

Research has shown that numerous adverse events affecting patient safety are associated with insufficient consideration of Human Factors and Ergonomics (HFE) in the development and execution of technologies, processes, workflows, job roles, teams, and socio-technical systems. In recent years, HFE has gained prominence as an essential field focused on minimizing medication errors, enhancing the design and application of Health Information Technology (HIT), and mitigating risks that could result in patient falls [12–15]. From an HFE perspective, patient safety activities should to not only aim reduce medical errors and enhance patient safety but also improve human well-being, job satisfaction, motivation, and technology acceptance by both patients and healthcare systems. For example, HFE principles suggest that patient safety enhancement programs that increase the workload of healthcare personnel are not justifiable and should not be implemented, as this could indirectly lead to negative effects over time due to the increased burden on staff [16].

1.3 The role of human factors in preventing medical errors

Medical errors often stem from complex, multifactorial issues where human performance plays a critical role. By understanding human limitations, such as attention lapses, cognitive overload, and fatigue, interventions can be designed to mitigate these risks. For instance, introducing standardized procedures, optimizing work environments, and improving team communication can create conditions that are less prone to error [17].

Several studies have shown that a significant proportion of medical errors are preventable [18–20]. According to Reason's Swiss Cheese Model [21], errors occur when multiple layers of defense are breached due to system flaws and human factors aligning. By addressing these factors, healthcare providers can close gaps in the system that lead to harm. Incorporating human factors into healthcare can significantly reduce the likelihood of errors by improving the design of systems and processes, enhancing communication, and supporting healthcare workers' physical and mental capacities [22].

1.4 Importance of the chapter

This chapter aims to contribute to the existing body of knowledge by exploring how human factors directly influence the occurrence of errors in healthcare and providing evidence-based recommendations to mitigate these risks. It will also review models and strategies employed in other high-stakes industries, such as aviation, and examine how they can be adapted to healthcare settings.

2. Types of medical errors

Healthcare professionals need to be aware of the various types of medical errors to gain a clearer understanding of the adverse events that may arise. By pinpointing the shortcomings, failures, and risk factors that contribute to these events, corrective actions can be formulated to prevent similar mistakes in the future. Consequently, all individuals involved in healthcare can assist in implementing effective preventative strategies aimed at minimizing future medical errors and enhancing patient safety. The following are the types of medical errors that are of greater significance [23].

2.1 Diagnostic errors

Diagnostic errors occur when a healthcare provider fails to accurately identify a patient's condition. These errors include delayed diagnosis, misdiagnosis, or complete failure to diagnose. Studies estimate that diagnostic errors account for approximately 10–15% of all medical errors and are a leading cause of malpractice claims globally.

Example: A patient presenting with chest pain may be diagnosed with a less severe condition, such as heartburn, instead of a life-threatening condition like a myocardial infarction. The delay in appropriate treatment could result in severe consequences, including death.

2.1.1 Contributing human factors

Cognitive bias: Physicians may rely on heuristics (mental shortcuts) leading to confirmation bias or anchoring bias, where they stick to an initial diagnosis despite new evidence.

Time pressure: Diagnostic errors are more common in high-pressure, busy environments where physicians are rushed.

2.2 Medication errors

Medication errors include mistakes in prescribing, dispensing, or administering medication. These errors can result in adverse drug events (ADEs), which cause harm to patients. Studies suggest that 1 in 10 patients in developed countries experience a medication-related injury each year, many of which are preventable.

Example: A nurse administering 10 mg of a medication instead of the prescribed 1 mg due to a misplaced decimal point in the order. This dosing error can cause serious, even fatal, consequences.

2.2.1 Contributing human factors

Poorly designed electronic health records (EHRs): Confusing or cluttered interfaces can lead to incorrect entries.

Communication breakdowns: Failure to properly convey dosage information between healthcare providers can result in wrong medications being administered.

2.3 Surgical errors

Surgical errors, or "never events," are mistakes that should never happen in an operating room. These include wrong-site surgery, operating on the wrong patient, leaving surgical instruments inside the body, and anesthesia-related errors.

Example: Performing surgery on the wrong limb or organ due to inadequate pre-surgical marking or team verification can have devastating and irreversible outcomes.

2.3.1 Contributing human factors

Team communication failures: Miscommunication between surgeons, anesthetists, and nursing staff can lead to catastrophic mistakes.

Fatigue: Surgeons and staff working extended hours or overnight shifts are more prone to errors.

2.4 Communication errors

Communication errors often occur during transitions in patient care, such as handoffs between shifts or transfers between departments. These errors can lead to incomplete or incorrect information being passed along, increasing the likelihood of adverse events.

Example: During a shift change in an ICU, a critical piece of information about a patient's allergy is omitted, leading to the administration of a drug that causes an allergic reaction.

2.4.1 Contributing human factors

Ineffective handoff processes: A lack of standardized communication protocols or checklists increases the risk of missed information.

Assumptions: Healthcare providers might assume that certain information is already known by their colleagues, leading to gaps in care.

2.5 System and process errors

System errors refer to failures in organizational processes or workflows that make it difficult for healthcare professionals to perform their duties safely. These errors may involve faulty equipment, poorly designed healthcare processes, or inadequate staffing levels.

Example: A hospital's EHR system crashes frequently, forcing clinicians to rely on manual documentation, which increases the chance of transcription errors and miscommunication.

2.5.1 Contributing human factors

Complexity of healthcare systems: Overly complex workflows, equipment interfaces, or software systems increase the cognitive load on healthcare professionals.

Inadequate training: Without proper training on complex systems, healthcare workers are more likely to make errors when using new technologies.

2.6 Human performance errors

Human performance errors are typically associated with lapses in judgment, attention, or memory. These errors can be classified into slips (unintended actions), lapses (memory failures), and mistakes (errors in planning).

Example: A nurse intending to administer medication to patient A accidentally gives it to patient B due to momentary distraction or failure to double-check patient identity.

2.6.1 Contributing human factors

Cognitive overload: Multitasking and managing several patients simultaneously can lead to attention slips.

Fatigue: Long shifts without adequate breaks can result in diminished attention and impaired decision-making.

2.7 Summary of the sub-section

This sub-section has provided an overview of different types of medical errors and the role that human factors play in their occurrence. Whether it is diagnostic errors due to cognitive bias, medication errors from communication breakdowns, or system errors caused by poorly designed workflows, each type of error is linked to various human and system-related factors. Understanding these connections is crucial in designing effective interventions to reduce errors and improve patient safety.

3. The role of human factors in medical errors

Medical errors remain a significant challenge in healthcare, leading to adverse patient outcomes, increased healthcare costs, and a loss of trust in medical systems. Understanding the role of human factors in these errors is crucial for developing effective strategies to mitigate risks and improve patient safety. This sub-section explores the various ways human factors contribute to medical errors, highlighting key concepts, examples, and implications for practice.

3.1 Definition of human factors

Human factors refer to the study of how people interact with systems, tools, and environments. In healthcare, this includes understanding how healthcare professionals, patients, and technologies interact, as well as how cognitive, physical, and organizational factors influence behavior and decision-making [16].

Understanding human factors that contribute to medical errors is crucial for improving patient safety. Analyzing various models of human factors is essential in this context. The study of human error in the workplace, particularly from the perspectives of safety and human factors engineering, is not a new topic. Researchers have explored it through various models, highlighting its significance in healthcare. For example, James Reason has suggested that errors occur at four levels: (1) Unsafe Acts, which stem from operator activities; (2) Preconditions for Unsafe Acts, indicating the environmental factors involved in errors; (3) Supervisory Errors, which reflect managerial activities that influence operators; and (4) Organizational Influences, representing the culture, policies, and procedures that affect operators [21, 24]. According to Reason's perspective, humans are inherently prone to error, and systemic processes are often impacted by latent weaknesses [25]. In the following, we will examine causation models and the analysis of medical errors from the perspective of human factors to clarify the role of these factors in medical errors. Various models and frameworks help elucidate the complex interactions between human behavior, system design, and environmental factors.

3.2 Swiss cheese model

The Swiss Cheese Model (SCM), conceptualized by James Reason [26], serves as a vital framework for understanding the multifaceted nature of medical errors in healthcare settings (**Figure 1**). This model illustrates how errors can occur when multiple layers of defense fail to prevent adverse events. Each layer represents a safeguard—such as protocols, training, and technology—designed to mitigate risks. However, when the "holes" in these layers, which symbolize weaknesses or failures,

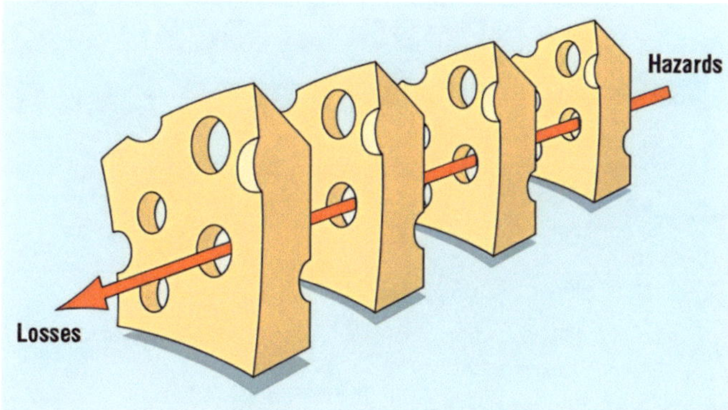

Figure 1.
Original Swiss cheese model (SCM).

align, the likelihood of an error reaching the patient increases significantly. This model identifies unsafe acts as the primary and direct cause of incidents and traces the origins of these unsafe acts across three levels: preconditions for unsafe acts, unsafe supervision, and organizational influences. According to this model, an incident will only occur when the holes present in the layers align. Furthermore, this model first introduces undesirable human actions as a cause of incidents and second emphasizes the role of factors and organizational deficiencies at various levels in shaping such actions within the workplace. At its core, the SCM emphasizes that no single factor is solely responsible for medical errors; rather, it is the convergence of multiple failures that leads to adverse events [26].

For instance, cognitive overload among healthcare providers can impair decision-making and attention. Stressful conditions and time constraints can exacerbate these cognitive challenges, creating an environment where errors are more likely to occur. Training deficiencies also contribute to the alignment of holes in this model. If healthcare professionals lack adequate training on protocols or equipment usage, their ability to navigate complex clinical situations diminishes. This lack of preparedness can create gaps that align with other systemic vulnerabilities. Organizational culture plays a crucial role in the effectiveness of the SCM. A culture that promotes open communication and encourages reporting of near misses fosters an environment where learning from errors is prioritized. Conversely, a blame-oriented culture may discourage staff from reporting mistakes or unsafe conditions, allowing holes in the cheese to go unaddressed. Leadership commitment is another essential element. When management prioritizes patient safety and allocates resources toward training and system improvements, it strengthens the layers of defense against medical errors. This proactive approach helps minimize the alignment of holes across different layers [27].

The SCM has been widely adopted in risk management strategies within healthcare [28–32]. By systematically analyzing incidents through this lens, organizations can identify specific vulnerabilities and implement targeted interventions. For example, after a medication error occurs, a thorough investigation using the SCM can reveal whether inadequate training, poor communication among staff, or insufficient protocols contributed to the incident. Furthermore, this model encourages continuous improvement by highlighting that defenses should not be static. Regular assessments and updates to training programs and protocols are essential to ensure that new vulnerabilities do not emerge as healthcare practices evolve [31].

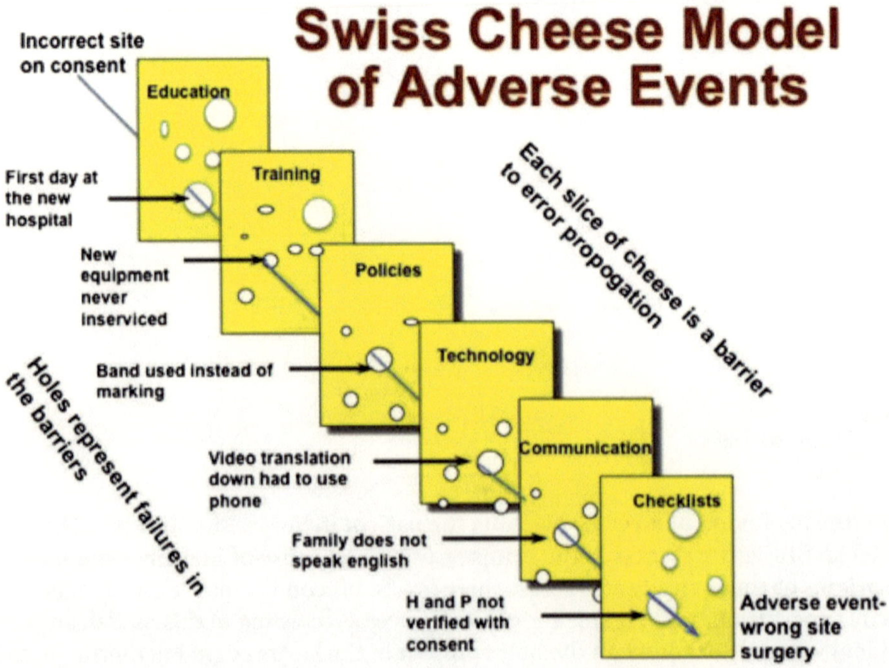

Figure 2.
Example of using the SCM to find the cause of wrong site surgery [27].

In summary, the SCM provides a comprehensive framework for understanding how human factors contribute to medical errors. By recognizing that errors result from a combination of individual actions and systemic failures, healthcare organizations can implement more effective strategies for prevention and risk management. Emphasizing training, fostering a supportive culture, and ensuring robust communication are key steps toward closing the gaps in defenses and enhancing patient safety in healthcare settings. This holistic approach not only aids in mitigating current risks but also prepares organizations for future challenges in patient care. An example of using the SCM to find the cause of an adverse event (wrong site surgery) is presented in **Figure 2**.

3.3 Human factors analysis and classification system (HFACS)

While the SCM by Reason provides a traditional framework for investigating incidents, it lacks the necessary characteristics for practical application in real-world scenarios. Specifically, the model struggles to accurately identify the precise nature of the holes in its layers. This limitation means that the types of failures occurring at each level are not fully detailed, rendering the model less practical. For the SCM to be systematically and effectively utilized as an analytical tool, the holes within the layers must be clearly defined. Without this clarity, the model falls short in addressing the complexities of human factors and their influence on medical errors [25].

To address the limitations of the SCM, Chapel and Wigman introduced the "Human Factor Classification and Analysis System (HFACS)" as a means to connect theoretical concepts with practical applications. The HFACS approach is specifically tailored to identify both latent and active flaws within the SCM, serving as an effective research tool [24].

HFACS is a widely utilized framework for examining human factors related to accidents in various sectors, such as aviation, railways, maritime, mining, manufacturing, and healthcare [25, 33–36]. This system is organized into causal categories aligned with Reason's four levels of error causation. Each category contains nanocodes that denote specific human behaviors or situational factors that may contribute to errors. By systematically identifying the causes of an adverse event and assigning them to one or more nanocodes, HFACS standardizes the investigative process and facilitates a thorough analysis of common factors leading to adverse events [24]. The HFACS framework is structured hierarchically into four main levels: unsafe acts, preconditions for unsafe acts, unsafe supervision, and organizational influences. Each level builds on the preceding one, tracing the reasons for errors from active to latent conditions, moving from unsafe acts to broader organizational influences. Within these four levels, there are 19 causal categories, which are illustrated in **Figure 3** (white boxes) and summarized in **Table 1** [37].

Recently, a modified version of the Human Factors Analysis and Classification System (HFACS) specifically designed for the causation and analysis of medical errors has been introduced by Jalali and colleagues [38]. In this model, also called HFACS-MEs, the causal levels have been expanded to five, with significant changes made to the categories within each level. Validation of this model for analyzing medical errors has also been conducted. The revised structure is illustrated in **Figure 4**, where the gray boxes indicate the modified or newly added causal categories. This expansion aims to provide a more comprehensive framework for identifying and understanding the complexities of medical errors, addressing some limitations found in the original HFACS model. The addition of a fifth causal level allows for a broader exploration of

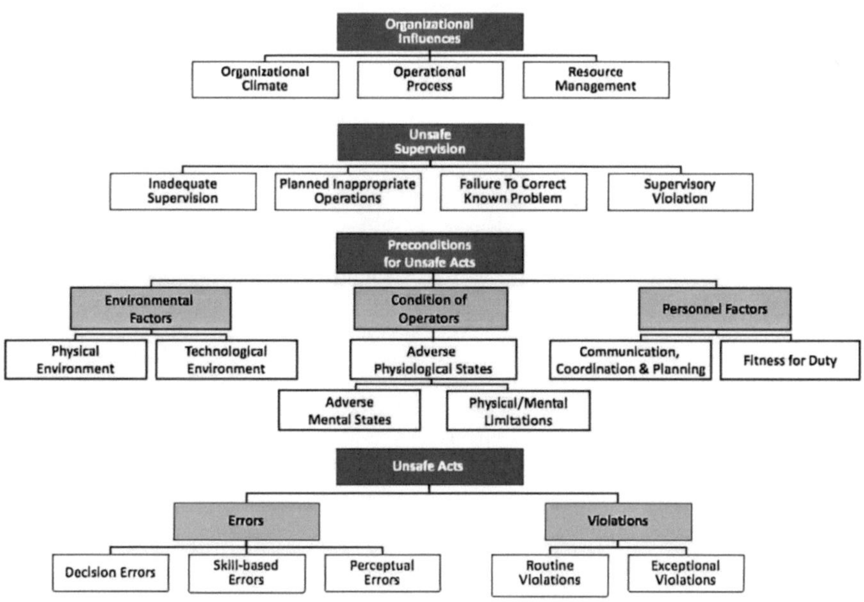

Figure 3.
The human factors analysis and classification system (HFACS) framework.

Organizational influences
Organizational climate: The overall environment or perspective within the organization, which encompasses elements like policies, command hierarchy, and cultural aspects. *Operational process*: The structured methodology through which an organization implements its vision, including operations, procedures, and supervision, among other factors. *Resource management*: The administration of essential resources, including human capital, financial assets, and equipment.
Unsafe supervision
Inadequate supervision: This refers to the insufficient oversight and management of personnel and resources. It encompasses factors such as training, professional support, and operational leadership, among others. *Planned inappropriate operations*: This involves the management and allocation of tasks, taking into account risk management, crew pairing, operational pace, and similar considerations. *Failed to correct known problems*: These are instances where supervisors are aware of deficiencies related to individuals, equipment, training, or other safety-related areas but allow these issues to persist without taking corrective action. *Supervisory violations*: This pertains to the intentional disregard for established rules, regulations, guidelines, or standard operating procedures by management while fulfilling their responsibilities.
Preconditions for unsafe acts
Environmental factors *Technological environment:* This category includes various aspects such as equipment and control design, display/interface features, checklist formats, task-related factors, and levels of automation. *Physical environment:* This encompasses the operational context, including elements like weather, altitude, and terrain, as well as ambient conditions such as heat, vibration, lighting, and the presence of toxins. *Conditions of the operator* *Adverse mental states:* These refer to acute psychological or mental conditions that impair performance, including mental fatigue, negative attitudes, and misplaced motivations. *Adverse physiological states:* This includes acute medical or physiological issues that hinder safe operations, such as illness, intoxication, and various pharmacological or medical conditions known to affect performance. *Physical/mental limitations:* These are permanent physical or mental disabilities that may negatively impact performance, including poor eyesight, lack of physical strength, limited mental capability, and chronic mental health issues. *Personnel factors* *Communication, coordination, and planning:* This involves various issues related to communication, teamwork, and coordination that can influence performance. *Fitness for duty:* This refers to off-duty behaviors necessary for optimal job performance, such as adhering to crew rest guidelines, alcohol restrictions, and other requirements for off-duty conduct.
Unsafe acts
Errors *Decision errors:* These errors, characterized as "thinking" mistakes, occur when planned actions are carried out as intended, yet the strategy proves insufficient or unsuitable for the circumstances. They often manifest in the form of poorly executed procedures, inappropriate choices, or the misinterpretation and misuse of relevant information. *Skill-based errors:* These are actions that have been practiced to the point of becoming automatic, occurring with little or no conscious awareness. Such "doing" errors may include breakdowns in visual scanning patterns, unintended activation or deactivation of controls, forgotten tasks, and omitted items in checklists. Even the method or technique employed while performing a task can be a source of these errors. *Perceptual errors:* These occur when sensory input is compromised, which is common when flying at night, in adverse weather, or in visually challenging environments. When faced with incomplete or unclear information, aircrew may misjudge distances, altitudes, and descent rates, and they may respond incorrectly to various visual or vestibular illusions. *Violations* *Routine violations:* Often referred to as "bending the rules," these violations tend to be habitual and are frequently tolerated by supervisors or management, allowing for deviations from established procedures. *Exceptional violations:* These are isolated incidents of deviation from authority that are not characteristic of the individual and are not approved by management.

Table 1.
Description of the HFACS categories.

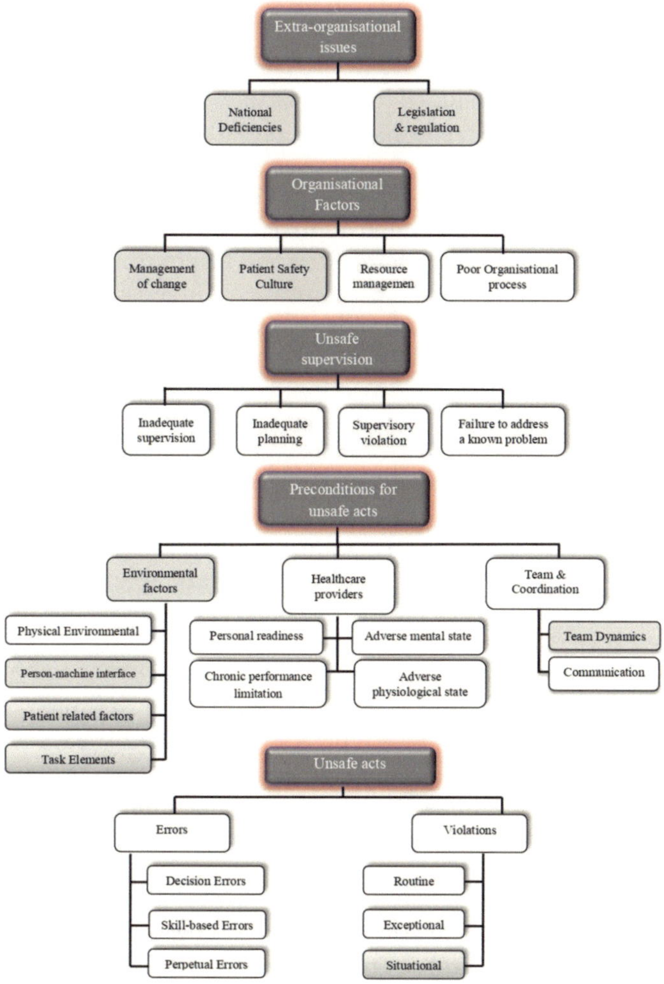

Figure 4.
New framework of the proposed human factors analysis and classification system for the medical errors (HFACS-MEs).

factors influencing medical errors, including those that extend beyond organizational boundaries. This is crucial for understanding how external influences can impact patient safety. The modifications made to the categories within each level enhance the model's ability to capture specific deficiencies that may contribute to errors, thus facilitating a more nuanced analysis. Validation studies have confirmed that this adapted HFACS model is effective in analyzing medical errors, making it a valuable tool for healthcare professionals seeking to improve safety outcomes. By providing a structured approach to identifying both latent and active failures, this model can help organizations develop targeted interventions to mitigate risks associated with medical errors. In summary, the newly developed HFACS model enhances the understanding of human factors in medical errors by providing a structured approach that integrates organizational influences and management roles into incident analysis. Its focus on identifying underlying causes rather than just individual mistakes allows for more effective interventions aimed at improving patient safety.

3.4 Systems engineering initiative for patient safety (SEIPS) model

The Systems Engineering Initiative for Patient Safety (SEIPS) Model is a comprehensive framework designed to enhance patient safety through systematic approaches. Developed by Carayon and colleagues, the SEIPS Model integrates various components of healthcare systems, emphasizing the interplay between people, tasks, tools, and the environment [39]. It identifies key elements that influence patient safety and provides a structured approach to analyze these components. The model highlights people, focusing on the roles and responsibilities of healthcare providers, patients, and families in the care process. Understanding how individuals interact within the system is crucial for identifying potential safety issues. Tasks refer to the activities performed within healthcare settings, including clinical procedures, documentation, and communication; analyzing these tasks helps identify inefficiencies or errors that could compromise patient safety. The tools and technology component encompasses all instruments and technologies used in patient care, from electronic health records to medical devices, as their effectiveness and usability significantly impact how safely tasks are performed. The environment plays a vital role in patient safety by considering the physical and organizational context in which care is delivered; factors such as layout, workflow, and policies can either facilitate or hinder safe practices. Finally, the model emphasizes the importance of measuring outcomes related to patient safety, including adverse events and overall quality of care.

The SEIPS Model can be applied in various ways to enhance patient safety: Organizations can use it to assess current practices by evaluating each component's contribution to safety; it aids in designing targeted interventions that address specific safety issues; and it serves as a framework for developing training programs that emphasize teamwork, communication, and effective use of technology [40]. Numerous studies have demonstrated the effectiveness of the SEIPS Model in real-world settings; for instance, hospitals implementing SEIPS-based interventions reported reductions in medication errors and improved communication among staff members [41]. These case studies underline the model's practical applicability in enhancing patient safety through systemic changes [42]. The SEIPS Model represents a paradigm shift in how healthcare organizations approach patient safety by focusing on systemic interactions rather than isolated incidents. It provides a robust framework for understanding and improving safety outcomes in complex healthcare environments. Future research should continue to explore its applications across diverse settings and populations to further validate its effectiveness. In summary, the SEIPS Model offers a structured approach to enhancing patient safety by considering multiple interrelated components within healthcare systems, leading to significant improvements in both clinical outcomes and overall care quality [43]. The framework of this model is presented in **Figure 5**.

3.5 Root cause analysis (RCA)

Root Cause Analysis (RCA) is a systematic method widely employed in healthcare to identify the underlying causes of medical errors. Its application is critical for enhancing patient safety and improving overall care quality. By delving into the root causes of errors, RCA facilitates a deeper understanding of the systemic issues that contribute to adverse events, ultimately guiding effective prevention strategies. The RCA process typically involves several key steps: defining the problem, collecting

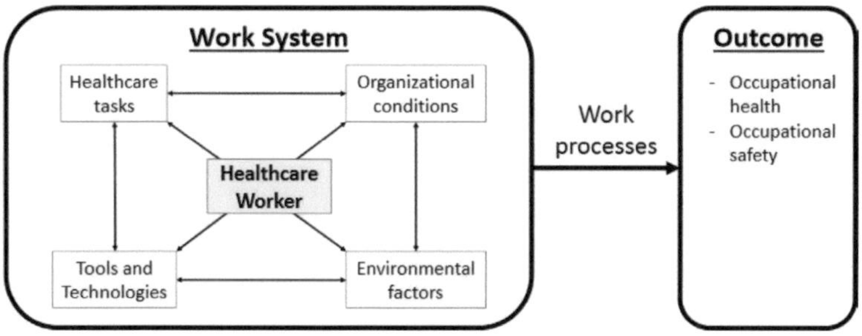

Figure 5.
Framework of systems engineering initiative for patient safety (SEIPS) model [44].

data, identifying contributing factors, analyzing root causes, developing recommendations, implementing solutions, and monitoring outcomes. This structured approach allows healthcare organizations to move beyond surface-level symptoms and focus on systemic issues that lead to errors [45].

For example, a study highlighted the successful use of RCA in American hospitals to improve safety and quality of care by addressing system defects rather than merely human errors. This approach not only helps identify specific incidents but also uncovers broader issues across various procedures, leading to simultaneous resolutions of multiple problems [46]. Another application of RCA was observed in an analysis of sentinel events in healthcare settings. This analysis revealed that many problems were related to care delivery issues, with a notable percentage stemming from knowledge and skill deficits among staff. By classifying these root causes, healthcare teams could implement tailored training programs aimed at addressing specific weaknesses [47]. RCA has also been effective in identifying communication failures within healthcare teams. A qualitative study found that many adverse events were linked to verbal communication errors during handovers and teamwork. Recognizing these communication gaps prompted organizations to develop improved protocols and training focused on effective communication strategies [48].

A key tool in this process is the Fishbone Diagram, which visually categorizes potential causes into distinct branches, such as people, processes, equipment, and environment. This structured approach helps teams systematically explore various factors contributing to errors [49]. For instance, in analyzing medication administration errors, a Fishbone Diagram can reveal issues like inadequate staff training and communication breakdowns as significant contributors [50]. A Fishbone Root Cause Analysis Diagram is presented in **Figure 6**.

Despite its strengths, RCA has several limitations and shortcomings that can affect its efficacy in addressing medical errors [51]. One significant issue is underreporting; RCA often relies on voluntary reporting of incidents, which can lead to incomplete data. Many healthcare professionals may hesitate to report errors due to fear of punitive consequences or an organizational culture that does not support transparency. Additionally, there is a potential for bias in the analysis process. If the team conducting the RCA has preconceived notions about the causes of an error, it may lead to overlooking critical factors or misattributing blame. Furthermore, while RCA aims to identify systemic issues, there is a tendency for some analyses to focus on individual mistakes rather than broader organizational factors, resulting in recommendations that do not effectively address root causes. Conducting thorough RCAs can also be resource-intensive, requiring significant time and effort from healthcare staff.

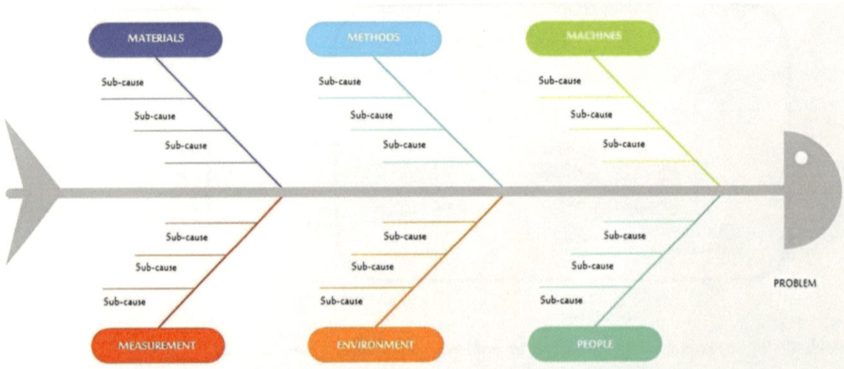

Figure 6.
Fishbone root cause analysis diagram.

In busy clinical environments, this can pose challenges in dedicating sufficient resources for comprehensive analysis. Moreover, implementing recommendations from RCA findings does not always occur effectively; organizations may struggle with follow-through on proposed changes due to competing priorities or lack of accountability. Lastly, the intricate nature of healthcare systems means that errors often arise from multiple interrelated factors. Traditional RCA techniques may struggle to capture this complexity fully, leading to oversimplified conclusions [52, 53].

In conclusion, Root Cause Analysis serves as a vital tool for identifying the underlying causes of medical errors in healthcare settings. By systematically analyzing incidents and understanding their root causes, organizations can implement effective strategies that enhance patient safety and reduce the likelihood of future errors. However, it is essential to acknowledge the limitations and shortcomings associated with RCA to ensure that its application leads to meaningful improvements in healthcare processes and culture. Addressing these challenges requires fostering a culture of safety where staffs feel empowered to report errors without fear and ensuring robust follow-up on recommendations derived from RCA findings.

3.6 Comparison of human factor methods in medical error analysis

RCA, HFACS, SEIPS, and SCM are all prominent methods used to analyze human factors and medical errors in healthcare. Each method offers unique perspectives and approaches to understanding and mitigating errors, but they also have distinct strengths and limitations. RCA is a traditional method focused on identifying the fundamental causes of adverse events. It typically follows a linear process that includes defining the problem, collecting data, identifying contributing factors, and developing recommendations. While RCA is widely used, it has been criticized for its lack of standardization across organizations and its tendency to focus on individual errors rather than systemic issues. Studies have shown that RCA often overlooks broader organizational factors that contribute to errors, which can limit its effectiveness in preventing future incidents [45, 54]. HFACS builds upon the foundations of RCA by providing a more structured framework for analyzing human error. HFACS categorizes errors into four levels: unsafe acts, preconditions for unsafe acts, unsafe supervision, and organizational influences. This comprehensive approach allows for a more nuanced understanding of how various human factors contribute to medical errors. Research indicates that HFACS can effectively aggregate data from multiple incidents, leading to actionable insights that enhance safety risk identification and assessment systems. Its systematic nature makes it more reliable than traditional RCA methods [24, 25, 55]. SEIPS Model emphasizes the interplay between people, tasks, tools, and the environment in healthcare settings. This model focuses on understanding how these components interact to influence patient safety outcomes. SEIPS encourages a holistic view of healthcare processes, making it valuable for identifying systemic issues that contribute to errors. However, while SEIPS offers a broad perspective on safety improvement, it may lack the detailed categorization of human errors found in HFACS [56]. SCM is a metaphorical framework used to illustrate how multiple layers of defense can prevent errors from resulting in adverse outcomes. Each layer represents a safeguard against failure; however, when holes (representing weaknesses) align across these layers, an error can occur. This model effectively highlights the importance of multiple defenses in risk management but tends to oversimplify complex interactions within healthcare systems [21]. While the SCM provides a traditional framework for investigating incidents, it lacks the necessary characteristics for practical application in real-world scenarios. Specifically, the model struggles to accurately identify the precise nature of the holes in its layers [25].

3.7 Conclusion

In summary, while all four methods—RCA, HFACS, SEIPS, and SCM—contribute valuable insights into human factors and medical error analysis, the HFACS method stands out as the most comprehensive and accurate approach. Its structured framework allows for detailed categorization of errors at multiple levels, facilitating a deeper understanding of how various human factors interact within healthcare systems. By addressing both individual actions and organizational influences, HFACS provides a more holistic view that can lead to effective interventions aimed at improving patient safety.

4. Strategies for reducing medical errors through human factors

Implementing effective strategies that focus on human factors can significantly reduce medical errors in healthcare settings. The best approach to reducing medical errors is to focus on the causal levels and categories in human factors analysis models [57]. For instance, after identifying the causes of medical errors using models like HFACS, paying attention to the levels and categories that play a significant role in the occurrence of these errors can enhance the effectiveness of interventions and make them more targeted. For example, the HFACS method has been applied in various hospital settings to identify the causes of medical errors, particularly in anesthesia, surgery, medication, trauma, and emergency departments [55]. In surgical processes, it is found that most errors were related to preconditions for unsafe acts, such as mental states, communication, coordination and technological environment. Unsafe supervision is another category of errors that have been reported in surgical process. In other hand, HFACS revealed that organizational factors played a major role in medication errors. In trauma and emergency departments, improper human resource management and decision-making were significant contributors to errors. Across all hospital settings, HFACS consistently identified preconditions for unsafe acts as the primary cause of medical incidents, such as communication failures, adverse mental states, and environmental factors [55]. HFACS has proven to be a reliable tool for pinpointing errors, enabling hospital managers to target interventions aimed at reducing human, supervisory, and organizational factors leading to medical errors.

As is evident, the HFACS model can identify various causal levels, both hidden and explicit, that contribute to medical errors. The main advantage of this approach lies in its attention to detail. Unlike methods such as RCA and the Swiss cheese model, HFACS precisely identifies the causes of errors through predefined nano-codes. This means it not only detects causal levels but also specifies, in full detail, the types of deficiencies occurring at each level. This strength highlights the model's practical applicability in identifying the causes of medical errors. In other words, HFACS is specifically designed to define both latent and active internal deficiencies within the Swiss cheese model, making it a suitable tool for systematic root cause analysis. This framework has been described and evaluated in hundreds of incident reports. The main distinction between HFACS and other accident causation models is that HFACS emphasizes the role of management and organizational factors as integral parts of the safety system. Its key advantage is that, rather than focusing on what mistake an individual made, it aims to deeply understand why the error occurred.

Currently, various approaches are used across different countries for recording, analyzing, and reducing medical errors, all aimed at the ultimate goal of preventing these errors. For example, in Iran, the RCA Committee, operating under the Patient Safety Administration, is responsible for reviewing and analyzing medical errors. In this committee, a team of specialists makes decisions regarding incidents that have occurred. The primary tool used in these committees for analyzing adverse medical events is the RCA method, which identifies the root causes of these incidents. In the United States, the Joint Commission requires that all serious patient harm events undergo a comprehensive RCA to determine why the event occurred and how similar events can be prevented in the future [58]. Unfortunately, traditional RCA has not proven effective in improving patient safety, as evidenced by the recurrence of similar harmful events even after RCA completion [59, 60].

The issue lies in the fact that traditional RCA does not effectively address human error as a primary cause of patient harm events. Instead, RCA is an engineering-based method rooted in the physical sciences, designed for uncovering causes of equipment failures and structural defects [61]. Traditional RCA methods often assume linear causality, where failures can be traced back to a single root cause [45]. This root cause can be discovered by asking a series of five "why" questions, with each answer forming the basis for the next question, ultimately leading to the root cause by the fifth question [62]. However, such methods and assumptions are not valid when applied to human error. Errors result from failures in complex, nonlinear interactions among tightly interconnected system variables, including human, environmental, task, technological, and organizational factors [43]. Thus, traditional RCA methods are inherently limited in reliably identifying why errors occur or how further harm from them can be prevented.

Given these shortcomings, the National Patient Safety Foundation released a set of guidelines known as Root Cause Analysis and Action, or RCA2 (pronounced "RCA squared") [58]. These guidelines assist users in transforming traditional RCA into a process focused on investigating and preventing harm associated with medical errors. Several changes to traditional RCA are included in these guidelines, such as employing RCA teams that are independent of the event, possess knowledge of human factors, and are specifically trained in conducting RCA. Other key changes include interviewing individuals involved in the event, developing causal/

contributory statements, identifying and implementing corrective actions, and engaging organizational leadership throughout the process. Unlike traditional RCA, RCA2 resembles a formal incident review process rather than an engineering failure analysis method. Indeed, the authors of RCA2 noted that these guidelines offer significant advancements in RCA investigations of patient harm events. However, these improvements are primarily focused on procedural changes in conducting RCA investigations and lack comprehensive guidance on analyzing human factors in patient harm events or implementing effective human factors interventions for systematically enhancing patient safety [8].

To address this critical gap, researchers have recently integrated a systematic complement of established human factors methods and tools into the RCA2 process. This process is based on the Human Factors Analysis and Classification System (HFACS) and the Human Factors Intervention Matrix (HFIX) [24, 63, 64]. By combining these methods with RCA2, researchers have developed a robust human factors process called HFACS-RCA2-HFIX, specifically designed to identify and prevent human factors and system-related issues associated with patient harm incidents [65]. The following sections will provide a description of the key human factors methods and tools used in this process, followed by a step-by-step overview of its overall structure.

4.1 Human factors frameworks, methods, and tools

4.1.1 The HFACS method

The Human Factors Analysis and Classification System (HFACS) framework is based on the theory of active and latent failures, widely recognized as the Swiss Cheese Model [66]. HFACS assumes that accidents and incidents are rarely linked to a single cause or contributing factor. Instead, they are often the result of multiple, interrelated factors interacting across four functional levels within an organization (see **Table 1**).

The first level pertains to unsafe acts by individuals directly involved in the incident, for instance, an emergency room doctor misdiagnosing appendicitis as gastroenteritis, or an ICU nurse failing to program an infusion pump. The second level, preconditions for unsafe acts, includes factors that can directly impact an individual's ability to perform tasks safely. Issues such as mental or physical fatigue, teamwork and communication challenges, technology design, and environmental conditions represent causal and contributory factors at this level.

Beyond individual and task conditions, the third level involves supervisory factors. Failures in supervisory oversight, excessive workload pressures, or lack of rule enforcement can lead to preconditions that contribute to unsafe acts. At the organizational level, factors such as safety culture, operational processes, and senior leadership decisions on resource allocation (such as funding, equipment, and personnel) can influence supervisors and preconditions that reinforce unsafe actions. A comprehensive description of the HFACS method, along with a new structure of this framework specifically adapted for analyzing medical errors (HFACS-MEs) as recently developed by Jalali et al. [38], is provided in Section 3.3.

During investigations of adverse medical events within RCA committees, HFACS and its associated tools (such as the HFACS interview guide and level-specific nanocodes) help facilitate the identification and analysis of multiple causal pathways across organizational layers that led to the event in question. By doing so, RCA committee members can reliably and comprehensively identify various opportunities for interventions to prevent event recurrence.

4.1.2 The HFIX method

While HFACS facilitates the identification of systemic issues that require attention, it does not support RCA investigators in determining how to address these issues. To aid this process, the HFIX method and its associated tools were developed to facilitate the identification of corrective actions following an HFACS analysis. HFIX is modeled after the Haddon Matrix [64], originally developed in the context of car accident/injury prevention. The HFIX tool assists users in thinking broadly and strategically about how to reduce risk by employing established safety science principles. When using HFIX, users align each HFACS causal pathway with five specific types of intervention approaches. Each approach represents strategies commonly used by safety professionals in various fields (e.g., systems engineering, behavioral sciences, and safety management). Through a series of questions or prompts, the HFIX tool enables users to systematically consider how each safety approach might translate into potential interventions to reduce risk.

The HFIX matrix aligns HFACS Level 1 (Unsafe Acts) with five different safety approaches (organizational/management-level intervention, personnel intervention, technology and equipment design intervention, task and mission intervention, and physical/operational environment intervention) and five evaluation criteria (feasibility, acceptability, cost, effectiveness, and durability) (**Figure 7**). Unsafe acts (such as medical errors or adverse medical events) performed by operators include five types: routine errors, exceptional errors, perception errors, decision errors, and skill-based errors. These unsafe acts can be mitigated through intervention approaches at the organizational/administrative level, personnel intervention, technology and equipment design intervention, task and mission intervention, and, finally, intervention in the physical/operational environment [64, 67].

4.1.3 HFACS-RCA2-HFIX process

In this process, human factors tools are integrated into various stages of the RCA2 process. These tools assist trained, interdisciplinary RCA teams in performing activities such as (1) gathering factual information through interviews with stakeholders

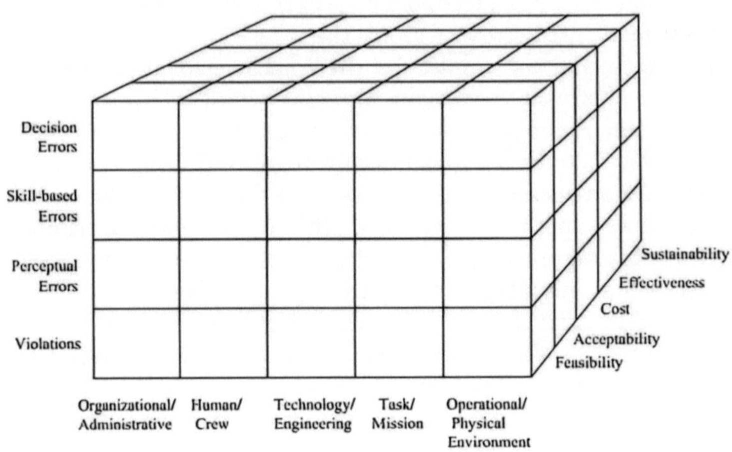

Figure 7.
Structure of the human factors intervention matrix (HFIX).

to determine what happened, (2) conducting cause-and-effect analyses to explain the reasons behind the event, and (3) formulating recommendations to prevent the recurrence of similar events. The HFACS-RCA2-HFIX process includes active support from senior leaders in the organization (i.e., executive sponsors), involvement of clinical stakeholders engaged in the patient harm event, and input from operational owners responsible for implementing changes, as well as interdisciplinary committees and safety, health, and risk management specialists overseeing the RCA process and the implementation of recommendations.

4.2 Process description

This process begins when a potential or actual patient safety event is identified and reported. The event report is then submitted to the event review committee. This committee consists of an interdisciplinary team of individuals with various areas of expertise (e.g., occupational safety and health specialists, clinical performance, organizational operations, quality management) who have been trained in the event review process. Safety and health experts, given their expertise in risk assessment and management, may take on a leadership role within this committee.

The members of the committee collaboratively review the report, the patient's electronic health record, and any other available information related to the event. They then utilize a standardized method to score the actual or potential severity of the event. For instance, they may use the risk matrix provided by the Joint Commission to identify significant events [58]. If the event exceeds the defined criteria levels, it will be selected to initiate the RCA process. Once this occurs, the committee chair activates the next steps in the HFACS-RCA2-HFIX process.

When the RCA for an event is initiated, a senior leader in the clinical area where the event occurred is identified and informed of this decision. This senior leader, who has been trained in the HFACS-RCA2-HFIX process and is aware of their roles and responsibilities, acts as the executive sponsor for the RCA. The executive sponsor is responsible for overseeing the RCA investigations and subsequent recommendations. The executive sponsor participates in the RCA process meetings and will be present throughout the process, providing guidance and support to the RCA team and ensuring that their administrative staffs are available to assist the RCA team with logistical, communication, and planning issues.

Upon initiating the RCA, the "on call" members of the RCA team are notified and activated. RCA teams consist of trained members, including physicians, nurses, occupational safety and health professionals acting as risk managers (RM), and quality improvement specialists (QIS). If necessary, the teams may also include trained and temporary members from other specialties. The designated facilitator for the RCA team is an RM or QIS who has experience in facilitating teams. After activation, the RCA facilitator utilizes their HFACS-RCA2-HFIX planning guide to gather initial information about the event and prepare for the team's first meeting.

The first meeting is held 3 to 5 days after the team is activated at a predetermined time on the RCA team members' calendars for the period during which they are "on call." During this meeting, the RCA team discusses what is known about the event. To determine the cause of the event, they develop an initial timeline of the event and gather additional factual information that aids in identifying its cause.

Next, the team identifies individuals they wish to interview and the objectives of these interviews. Using the HFACS-RCA2-HFIX interview guides and templates, they formulate specific questions focusing on human factors and systemic issues.

The responsibilities of the interviewers are then agreed upon by the team. Whenever possible, responsibilities are based on the clinical backgrounds of the RCA team members and the interviewees (e.g., nurses interviewing nurses, physicians interviewing physicians, pharmacists interviewing pharmacists). The team then postpones to carry out their designated activities.

Following Meeting 1, the RCA facilitator works with the administrative assistant of the executive sponsor to coordinate the timing and location of the interviews. If there are barriers to scheduling the interviews, the executive sponsor assists in guiding and resolving issues (e.g., freeing clinical duties for those being interviewed). During each interview, RCA team members utilize the interview questions developed by their team to structure the conversation around the HFACS-MEs framework. After the interviews, team members upload their notes to a shared folder on a secure server. This folder serves as a central repository for information related to the case, allowing team members to access and review materials before the next meeting.

The second meeting is typically held 2 weeks after Meeting 1. In this meeting, the RCA team members share insights gained from reviewing interview summaries and other information. Based on this review, they finalize the main timeline and establish "what" happened. Next, they use the HFACS-MEs framework and tools to structure their conversation around human factors and systemic issues and organize their thoughts about "why" the event occurred. They apply HFACS-MEs analysis tools to conduct a formal cause-and-effect analysis, identify critical causal pathways, and develop causal statements. Subsequently, they consider how to prevent the recurrence of this event and other similar events. Using HFIX tools, the team generates a list of potential solutions for the identified causal factors and selects their final recommendations based on these solutions.

During the third meeting, held about 1 week after Meeting 2, key stakeholders involved in the event and operational owners responsible for implementing changes meet with the RCA team and executive sponsor. Together, they discuss the team's findings and recommendations. These stakeholders then provide feedback to the RCA team, particularly regarding the types of changes recommended by the team (e.g., appropriateness, feasibility, potential barriers). The RCA team and executive sponsor use this feedback to prepare their report using the standard HFACS-RCA2-HFIX report template.

After Meeting 3, the RCA facilitator finalizes the team report and submits it to the RCA oversight committee for inclusion on the agenda for the next committee meeting. The members of this oversight committee include leadership stakeholders trained in the HFACS-RCA2-HFIX process from various clinical services within the organization. During the committee meeting, a summary of the RCA report is presented by a member of the RCA team, the executive sponsor, and operational owners of the proposed changes. The committee provides feedback on the appropriateness of the recommendations based on the RCA findings and their knowledge of past efforts to resolve similar issues. This committee also assists in identifying resources needed for implementing changes and developing strategies to facilitate execution.

Once the recommendations are approved, operational owners, with support from the executive sponsor, are responsible for implementing the changes. The RM or QIS who facilitated the RCA related to the change is also available for consultation and support as needed. However, they are not the owner of the change or responsible for carrying out the work. Operational owners are required to provide regular progress reports to the executive sponsor and the interdisciplinary patient safety committee that oversees quality improvement and safety efforts across the organization. Milestones are tracked by the safety manager and reported to this committee. The patient safety committee collaborates with the operational owner and executive sponsor to overcome barriers until changes are fully implemented. After the implementation process is completed, the patient safety committee and the patient safety officer monitor the effectiveness of the changes by tracking the recurrence of similar events. This information is then used to provide feedback to the RCA teams, executive sponsors, and the RCA oversight committee to inform their future RCA investigations. In this way, the HFACS-RCA2-HFIX process concludes with the root cause analysis of adverse medical events and the design and implementation of strategies for managing and mitigating these events.

The use of the HFACS-RCA2-HFIX process is one of the best approaches for identifying the causes of medical errors and implementing interventions to reduce these errors. This process has recently been implemented in an 18-month study at a large university health center in the western United States, and its success has been assessed [65]. The results of this case study demonstrated that the implementation of HFACS-RCA2-HFIX is feasible and more effective than traditional RCA in identifying and addressing the systemic causes of patient harm. The HFACS-RCA2-HFIX process provides a robust human factors framework for classifying, coding, and archiving causal factors in patient harm events. As a result, it offers healthcare risk managers the opportunity to analyze causal data at the level of the countries involved and to identify systemic trends in the various human factors that frequently lead to harm. Such data allows for clearer identification of system risks and makes it easier to justify the need for major changes in systems to reduce risk [68]. Furthermore, the ability to track the occurrence of different types of causal factors among events provides healthcare risk managers with the empirical data necessary to evaluate the effectiveness of their risk reduction efforts (i.e., return on investment). Such data is highly valuable when making decisions about strengthening or reallocating resources to various risk reduction efforts.

4.3 Some key approaches in reducing medical errors

A multifaceted approach that emphasizes teamwork, standardization, error reporting, technological integration, and continuous education is vital in promoting safety and enhancing the quality of care in healthcare systems. By prioritizing these strategies, healthcare organizations can significantly reduce the incidence of medical errors, ultimately leading to improved patient outcomes and a safer healthcare environment. In the rest of this chapter, some key approaches that can lead to the improvement of patient safety and quality of care are briefly presented.

4.3.1 Teamwork and communication training

Enhancing collaboration: Training programs focused on teamwork and communication emphasize the importance of collaboration among healthcare professionals. Effective interprofessional communication is crucial during patient handoffs and critical care situations.

Structured handoffs: Implementing standardized handoff protocols can minimize misunderstandings and ensure that essential patient information is accurately communicated.

Briefings and debriefings: Regular team briefings before procedures and debriefings afterward help clarify roles, expectations, and potential concerns, fostering a culture of shared responsibility and awareness.

Interventions for communication errors: Structured communication training targets decision errors and skill-based errors by encouraging clear information transfer and role clarification, minimizing misunderstandings that can lead to unsafe actions.

4.3.2 Standardization and protocols

Checklists for safety: The use of checklists in surgical procedures, medication administration, and other critical tasks has been shown to significantly reduce errors. Checklists help ensure that essential steps are not overlooked.

Standard operating procedures (SOPs): Establishing standardized procedures for common tasks helps eliminate variability in practice, reducing the likelihood of errors due to differing approaches among staff.

Guidelines and protocols: Developing clear, evidence-based guidelines for clinical practice provides a framework for decision-making, enhancing consistency and safety in patient care.

Interventions for decision and skill-based errors: Checklists and SOPs help prevent decision errors by providing structured steps; ensuring staff follow correct procedures while also addressing skill-based errors by reinforcing correct task execution.

4.3.3 Error reporting systems

Encouraging reporting: Implementing user-friendly error reporting systems encourages healthcare professionals to report near misses and errors without fear of punishment. This fosters a culture of transparency and learning.

Learning from mistakes: Analyzing reported errors allows organizations to identify trends and root causes, enabling targeted interventions to prevent recurrence.

Feedback mechanisms: Providing feedback to staff on reported incidents promotes accountability and reinforces the importance of error reporting as a tool for improving safety.

Interventions for routine and exceptional violations: A robust error reporting system helps identify routine violations (e.g., habitual bypassing of procedures) and exceptional violations (e.g., rare but egregious violations), allowing for focused corrective measures, such as retraining or revision of policies.

4.3.4 Simulation training

Realistic training environments: Simulation training provides healthcare professionals with opportunities to practice skills and decision-making in a safe, controlled environment. Scenarios can be tailored to reflect real-life challenges and high-pressure situations.

Team-based simulations: Conducting team-based simulations helps improve teamwork, communication, and coordination among healthcare providers, particularly in emergency situations.

Debriefing after simulations: Structured debriefings following simulations allow participants to reflect on their performance, discuss challenges, and identify areas for improvement.

Interventions for perceptual and skill-based errors: Simulations address perceptual errors (e.g., misjudging a patient's condition) and skill-based errors by replicating complex, high-stress scenarios, allowing healthcare workers to practice recognizing cues and refining their motor skills.

4.3.5 Technology integration

Electronic health records (EHRs) for improved accuracy: Implementing EHRs helps streamline documentation and reduces the risk of errors associated with handwritten notes. EHRs can facilitate accurate medication reconciliation and patient information access.

Decision support systems: Integrating clinical decision support tools within EHRs can provide real-time alerts for potential drug interactions, allergies, and other critical information, assisting clinicians in making informed decisions.

Automation and safety: Automation of routine tasks, such as medication dispensing and laboratory tests, reduces the likelihood of human error and enhances efficiency in patient care processes.

Interventions for decision and routine violations: EHRs and automated systems reduce decision errors by offering real-time clinical support and reduce routine violations by automating processes that might otherwise be bypassed due to time pressure or perceived irrelevance.

4.3.6 Intervention on preconditions for unsafe acts and unsafe acts

Managing fatigue and stress: Implementing workload management and staff rotation schedules can help reduce fatigue and stress, which are common preconditions for unsafe acts such as decision and skill-based errors. Regular mental health support and counseling for healthcare workers can mitigate emotional stress and improve decision-making.

Improving physical work environments: Optimizing the physical environment (e.g., lighting, ergonomics, and noise reduction) can reduce distractions and physical strain, leading to fewer perceptual errors and physical missteps.

Human factors engineering: Incorporating human factors engineering into healthcare processes can help design systems that reduce the likelihood of perceptual and skill-based errors by accounting for human limitations.

Prevention of routine and exceptional violations: Educating staff on the consequences of both routine violations (e.g., bypassing safety steps) and exceptional violations (e.g., rare, extreme deviations from protocol) helps foster a culture of safety and responsibility.

4.4 Case studies: Human factors in action

Examining real-world case studies can provide valuable insights into the impact of human factors on patient safety and medical errors. Here are three notable examples that illustrate both challenges and successful interventions in healthcare settings.

4.4.1 Case study 1: The impact of poor communication on patient outcomes

Background: In a busy urban hospital, a patient with a complex medical history was transferred from the intensive care unit (ICU) to a general ward. During the handoff, critical information regarding the patient's allergies and medication regimen was inadequately communicated between the nursing staff.

Incident: Shortly after the transfer, the patient was administered a medication that they were allergic to, resulting in a severe allergic reaction. The delay in identifying the reaction led to complications that extended the patient's hospital stay and increased healthcare costs.

4.4.2 Analysis

Communication breakdown: The handoff protocol was not followed, and there was a lack of structured communication tools (e.g., SBAR—Situation, Background, Assessment, and Recommendation).

Impact on outcomes: The incident highlighted how poor communication can lead to serious adverse events and emphasized the need for standardized handoff procedures.

4.4.3 Interventions

1. Implementation of a standardized handoff tool (SBAR) across the hospital.

2. Regular training sessions for staff on effective communication practices during patient transfers.

4.4.4 Case study 2: A successful implementation of checklists to reduce surgical errors

Background: A surgical department in a large academic medical center faced a high rate of surgical errors, including wrong-site surgeries and retained surgical instruments.

Intervention: The department adopted the World Health Organization (WHO) Surgical Safety Checklist, which includes critical safety checks before anesthesia, before incision, and before the patient leaves the operating room.

4.4.5 Analysis

Communication breakdown: The handoff protocol was not followed, and there was a lack of structured communication tools (e.g., SBAR—Situation, Background, Assessment, and Recommendation).

Impact on outcomes: The incident highlighted how poor communication can lead to serious adverse events and emphasized the need for standardized handoff procedures.

4.4.6 Results

1. A study conducted over 6 months showed a 40% reduction in surgical errors.

2. The implementation of the checklist also improved team communication and collaboration in the operating room.

4.4.7 Analysis

Standardization: The checklist provided a structured approach to ensure all necessary safety checks were completed, reducing variability in practice.

Team engagement: Involving the entire surgical team in the checklist process fostered a culture of safety and accountability.

Follow-up: The department continued to monitor surgical outcomes and refined the checklist based on staff feedback, further enhancing its effectiveness.

4.4.8 Case study 3: The role of fatigue management programs in reducing medical errors

Background: A regional hospital noted an increase in medication errors among nursing staff working long shifts, particularly during night shifts. Research indicated that fatigue significantly impacted alertness and performance.

Intervention: The hospital implemented a fatigue management program, which included: (1) education on the effects of fatigue on performance, (2) policies to limit the number of consecutive night shifts, and (3) provision of scheduled breaks and opportunities for power naps.

4.4.9 Results

1. Following the implementation of the program, there was a 30% decrease in medication errors reported by nursing staff.

2. Staff satisfaction and morale improved, leading to enhanced teamwork and communication.

4.4.10 Analysis

Awareness and training: Educating staff about the risks associated with fatigue fostered a greater understanding of its impact on patient safety.

Supportive environment: The program created a culture that prioritized staff well-being, recognizing the link between staff fatigue and patient outcomes.

Continued efforts: The hospital continues to monitor error rates and staff fatigue levels, making adjustments to the program as needed.

4.5 Conclusion

Reducing medical errors through human factors strategies is essential for improving patient safety and quality of care in healthcare settings. By prioritizing teamwork and communication training, implementing standardization and protocols, promoting error reporting, utilizing simulation training, and integrating technology, healthcare organizations can foster a culture of safety that minimizes risks and enhances overall outcomes. The expertise of occupational health and safety professionals is crucial in this process, as their specialized knowledge can guide the effective implementation of human factors approaches, ensuring that safety measures are both practical and tailored to the specific needs of the healthcare environment.

Utilizing the HFACS-RCA2-HFIX framework in identifying the root causes of medical errors and developing appropriate intervention strategies can significantly enhance prevention efforts. This comprehensive approach allows for a deeper understanding of the complexities involved in error occurrences, facilitating the design of targeted interventions that address both human and systemic factors. Continuous evaluation and adaptation of these strategies will ensure that they remain effective in an ever-evolving healthcare landscape. Additionally, the presented case studies demonstrate the vital role that human factors play in ensuring patient safety and highlight the effectiveness of targeted interventions. By focusing on communication, standardization through checklists, and addressing staff fatigue, healthcare organizations can significantly reduce medical errors and improve patient outcomes. The involvement of safety and health experts can further enhance these efforts by providing insights into the systemic factors that contribute to errors and identifying best practices for implementation. Continuous learning and adaptation based on real-world experiences, supported by the expertise of occupational health and safety professionals, will be key to advancing safety in healthcare settings.

5. The role of safety and health experts in reducing medical errors

In healthcare systems, the neglect of human factors in reducing medical errors has led to the exclusion of occupational safety and health experts from the analysis of adverse medical events. This has resulted in analyses often being conducted solely from a clinical perspective, overlooking the important and specialized role of safety and health experts in this field. Occupational safety and health play a fundamental role in preventing accidents and reducing errors in workplace environments, and this role can be particularly significant in the medical sector as well. This importance becomes more apparent when systematic analysis models like HFACS-MEs are utilized. This model examines the underlying causes of errors, including organizational, managerial, environmental, and individual factors, focusing on discovering the reasons behind the errors rather than just the outcomes.

The HFACS-MEs model aims to identify factors at various levels and analyze the complex interactions that influence unsafe practices in medical processes, thereby offering an approach that goes beyond traditional RCA and the main HFACS model. Such an approach not only aids in more accurately identifying error factors but also enables safety and health teams and physicians to implement intervention strategies tailored to environmental, human, and organizational conditions using tools like HFIX.

The role of occupational safety and health experts in monitoring and preventing medical errors is especially crucial in sensitive environments like hospitals. These experts contribute to creating safer environments and preventing the recurrence of similar errors by employing accident analysis tools and implementing risk management processes. By implementing models like HFACS-RCA2-HFIX, safety and health experts can take on a more active role as risk managers, leading to significant improvements in patient safety and a reduction in medical errors.

However, in many countries, traditional RCA processes often lack the involvement of these experts, viewing medical errors primarily from a clinical perspective. The use of more comprehensive analytical tools enhances the visibility of occupational safety and health experts' roles and aids in promoting safety within healthcare systems. Overall, the role of occupational safety and health experts in reducing medical errors and improving patient safety is essential and broad, yet unfortunately, it has not received serious attention in various countries. Safety and health experts working in hospitals and healthcare systems must not only identify and control hazardous factors but also effectively participate in the root cause analysis of medical errors and the design and implementation of effective interventions to reduce these errors by considering human factors. Collaboration between safety and risk management professionals and clinical experts within systematic processes like HFACS-RCA2-HFIX will contribute to the reduction of medical errors and the enhancement of patient safety. It is also important to note that safety and health experts need to increase their awareness and skills regarding human factors and their impact on medical errors to fulfill their roles effectively.

6. Limitations and future research needs

In this chapter, the aim has been to provide a comprehensive insight into medical errors and the role of human factors in identifying and reducing these errors. The role of safety and health experts in enhancing patient safety in healthcare facilities has also been thoroughly examined. However, this section of the book faces limitations that must be acknowledged. Since the foundation of reducing medical errors relies on accurate and precise root cause analysis, this chapter has introduced various methods and models used for this purpose. Nonetheless, the lack of comprehensive coverage of all existing models in the analysis of medical errors may relate to the constraints of the book's volume. Although the primary focus has been on HFACS and RCA2 models, other important methods in this field may have been overlooked. Furthermore, some concepts lean more on theoretical foundations and previous studies, and due to limitations in statistical data and empirical research, there may not be sufficient objective evidence to support them. Additionally, the models examined often pertain specifically to the healthcare systems of developed countries, and their implementation in other cultures and healthcare systems may encounter challenges.

Nonetheless, it is important to note that attention to human factors and the utilization of the expertise of occupational safety and health professionals in preventing medical errors are still in their early stages and require the development and testing of various models and processes. For future studies, research such as "Examining the Impact of Multi-Criteria Decision-Making (MCDM) Methods on Improving Medical Error Management Processes" and "Integrating Bayesian Networks, the HFACS-MEs Model, and HFIX (HFACS-BN-HFIX) for Root Cause Analysis and Strategy Development in Reducing Medical Errors" is recommended. Additionally, topics like "A Comparative Study of the Role of Organizational Culture in Preventing Medical Errors in Various Hospitals" and "Developing and Implementing Analytical Tools Based on Machine Learning Techniques for Identifying and Predicting Medical Errors" are also highly attractive.

It is essential to develop studies to determine the feasibility of implementing HFACS-RCA2-HFIX in other healthcare systems, especially smaller systems with limited resources. Furthermore, examining the impact of HFACS-RCA2-HFIX on quantitative outcomes, including data related to causal factors, recommendations, and the extent of patient harm, necessitates more detailed analyses that should be considered in future studies. Finally, a follow-up study to determine the sustainability of the HFACS-RCA2-HFIX approach is also critically needed.

7. Chapter conclusion

The analysis of human factors in medical errors remains a critical aspect of improving patient safety in healthcare systems. While models like the SCM, RCA, and SEIPS each offer valuable frameworks for understanding and mitigating errors, HFACS stands out as the most comprehensive and practical tool for identifying and addressing errors at multiple levels. The HFACS framework not only categorizes unsafe acts but also examines the underlying preconditions for these acts, such as environmental and cognitive factors, as well as the influence of inadequate supervision and broader organizational deficiencies. This layered approach allows for a more nuanced understanding of how different elements within the healthcare system interact to create conditions conducive to errors.

By systematically breaking down the causes of medical errors, HFACS facilitates the development of more effective, targeted interventions. These interventions go beyond simply addressing individual mistakes and instead focus on correcting systemic issues such as poor organizational oversight, inadequate training, communication failures, and environmental stressors. The structured nature of HFACS also allows for better aggregation and analysis of data, making it easier to identify recurring patterns and trends in medical errors across various healthcare settings.

Ultimately, the adoption of HFACS in healthcare organizations supports the creation of a culture of safety, where both human errors and systemic weaknesses are addressed comprehensively. By integrating HFACS into RCA and HFIX, healthcare providers can implement preventive strategies that reduce the likelihood of errors, enhance team communication, improve supervision, and optimize the design of healthcare environments. The expertise of occupational health and safety professionals is vital in this process; their specialized knowledge ensures that human factors approaches are implemented effectively, tailored to the specific needs of healthcare environments. This multifaceted approach to error prevention not only helps in mitigating immediate risks but also promotes long-term improvements in patient care, contributing to a safer and more reliable healthcare system. HFACS, with its ability to offer detailed insights into the interplay between human and organizational factors, is therefore indispensable for advancing patient safety initiatives and fostering a resilient healthcare culture that continuously evolves in response to emerging challenges.

Acknowledgements

The author acknowledges the use of ChatGPT for language correction and summarizing some of the sentences and paragraphs.

DOI: http://dx.doi.org/10.5772/intechopen.1008399

Author details

Mahdi Jalali
Neyshabur University of Medical Science, Neyshabur, Iran

*Address all correspondence to: jalalim1@nums.ac.ir

References

[1] Cohen TN. A human factors approach for identifying latent failures in healthcare settings [Doctor of Philosophy]. Daytona Beach, Florida: Embry-Riddle Aeronautical University; 2017

[2] Garrouste-Orgeas M, Philippart F, Bruel C, Max A, Lau N, Misset B. Overview of medical errors and adverse events. Annals of Intensive Care. 2012;**2**(1):1-9

[3] Vincent C. Patient safety. 2nd ed. Hoboken-USA: John Wiley & Sons; 2011

[4] Alemdar D, Yılmaz G. Evaluation of the relationship between the patient safety culture and medical error attitudes of the pediatric nurses. Clinical and Experimental Health Sciences. 2020;**10**(1):60-67

[5] Grober ED, Bohnen JMA. Defining medical error. Canadian Journal of Surgery. 2005;**48**(1):39

[6] Schwendimann R, Blatter C, Dhaini S, Simon M, Ausserhofer D. The occurrence, types, consequences and preventability of in-hospital adverse events–A scoping review. BMC Health Services Research. 2018;**18**:1-13

[7] Johnston BE, Lou-Meda R, Mendez S, Frush K, Milne J, Fitzgerald T. Teaching patient safety in global health: Lessons from the Duke Global Health patient safety fellowship. BMJ Global Health [Internet]. 2019;**4**(1):e001220. [Accessed: January 7, 2020]

[8] Organization WH. Global Patient Safety Action Plan 2021-2030: Towards Eliminating Avoidable Harm in Health Care. Geneva: World Health Organization; 2021

[9] Organization WH. Guidelines on Core Components of Infection Prevention and Control Programmes at the National and Acute Health Care Facility Level. Geneva: World Health Organization; 2016

[10] Sheikh A, Donaldson L, Dhingra-Kumar N, Bates D, Kelley E, Larizgoitia I. Patient Engagement: Technical Series on Safer Primary Care. Geneva: World Health Organization; 2016. p. 2016

[11] Carayon P, Wetterneck TB, Rivera-Rodriguez AJ, Hundt AS, Hoonakker P, Holden R, et al. Human factors systems approach to healthcare quality and patient safety. Applied Ergonomics. 2014;**45**(1):14-25

[12] Chou D. Health IT and patient safety: Building safer systems for better care. Journal of the American Medical Association. 2012;**308**(21):2282

[13] Holden RJ, Cornet VP, Valdez RS. Patient ergonomics: 10-year mapping review of patient-centered human factors. Applied Ergonomics. 2020;**82**:102972

[14] Hsieh MC, Chiang PY, Wang EMY, Kung WC, Hu YT, Huang MS, et al. The investigation of human error analysis in adverse drug events in Taiwan—From the perspective of causality assessment. Human Factors and Ergonomics in Manufacturing & Service Industries. 2019;**29**(4):340-349

[15] Kulich HR, Bass SR, Griscavage JS, Vijayvargiya A, Slowik JS, Koontz AM. An ergonomic comparison of three different patient transport chairs in a simulated hospital environment. Applied Ergonomics. 2020;**88**:103172

[16] Carayon P, Xie A, Kianfar S. Human factors and ergonomics as a patient

safety practice. BMJ Quality & Safety. 2014;**23**(3):196-205

[17] Taib IA, McIntosh AS, Caponecchia C, Baysari MT. A review of medical error taxonomies: A human factors perspective. Safety Science. 2011;**49**(5):607-615

[18] Northcott H, Vanderheyden L, Northcott J, Adair C, McBrien-Morrison C, Norton P, et al. Perceptions of preventable medical errors in Alberta, Canada. International Journal for Quality in Health Care. 2008;**20**(2):115-122

[19] Kumar S, Steinebach M. Eliminating US hospital medical errors. International Journal of Health Care Quality Assurance. 2008;**21**(5):444-471

[20] Merry AF, Anderson BJ. Medication errors–New approaches to prevention. Pediatric Anesthesia. 2011;**21**(7):743-753

[21] Reason J. Human error. New York: Cambridge University Press; 1990

[22] Kurniawan J, Duffy VG, editors. Systematic Review of the Importance of Human Factors in Incorporating Healthcare Automation. Midtown Manhattan, New York City: Springer; 2021

[23] Rodziewicz TLHB, Vaqar S, et al. Medical Error Reduction and Prevention. Treasure Island (FL): StatPearls Publishing; 2018. Available from: https://www.ncbi.nlm.nih.gov/books/NBK499956/ [Accessed: February 12, 2024]

[24] Shappell SA, Wiegmann DA. Applying Reason: The human factors analysis and classification system (HFACS). Human Factors and Aerospace Safety. 2001;**1**(1):59-86

[25] Diller T, Helmrich G, Dunning S, Cox S, Buchanan A, Shappell S. The human factors analysis classification system (HFACS) applied to health care. American Journal of Medical Quality. 2014;**29**(3):181-190

[26] Reason J, Hollnagel E, Paries J. Revisiting the Swiss cheese model of accidents. Journal of Clinical Engineering. 2006;**27**(4):110-115

[27] Seshia SS, Bryan Young G, Makhinson M, Smith PA, Stobart K, Croskerry P. Gating the holes in the Swiss cheese (part I): Expanding professor Reason's model for patient safety. Journal of Evaluation in Clinical Practice. 2018;**24**(1):187-197

[28] Bergeon F, Hensley M. Swiss cheese and the PRiMA model: What can information technology learn from aviation accidents? The Journal of Operational Risk. 2009;**4**(3):47

[29] Fukuoka K. Visualization of a hole and accident preventive measures based on the Swiss cheese model developed by risk management and process approach. WMU Journal of Maritime Affairs. 2016;**15**(1):127-142

[30] Fukuoka K, Furusho M. Relationship between latent conditions and the characteristics of holes in marine accidents based on the Swiss cheese model. WMU Journal of Maritime Affairs. 2016;**15**(2):267-292

[31] Kamoun F, Nicho M. Human and organizational factors of healthcare data breaches: The Swiss cheese model of data breach causation and prevention. International Journal of Healthcare Information Systems and Informatics (IJHISI). 2014;**9**(1):42-60

[32] Song W, Li J, Li H, Ming X. Human factors risk assessment: An integrated method for improving safety in clinical use of medical devices. Applied Soft Computing. 2020;**86**:105918

[33] Chen J-C, Chi C-F, Li W-C, editors. The analysis of safety recommendation and human error prevention strategies in flight operations. In: International Conference on Engineering Psychology and Cognitive Ergonomics. Midtown Manhattan, New York City: Springer; 2013

[34] Kilic B, Gümüş E. Application of HFACS to the nighttime aviation accidents and incidents. Journal of Aviation. 2020;**4**(2):10-16

[35] Li C, Tang T, Chatzimichailidou MM, Jun GT, Waterson P. A hybrid human and organisational analysis method for railway accidents based on STAMP-HFACS and human information processing. Applied Ergonomics. 2019;**79**:122-142

[36] Patterson JM, Shappell SA. Operator error and system deficiencies: Analysis of 508 mining incidents and accidents from Queensland, Australia using HFACS. Accident Analysis & Prevention. 2010;**42**(4):1379-1385

[37] Cohen TN. A human factors approach for identifying latent failures in healthcare settings [Doctor of Philosophy]. Daytona Beach, Florida: Embry-Riddle Aeronautical University; 2017

[38] Jalali M, Habibi E, Khakzad N, Aval SB, Dehghan H. A novel framework for human factors analysis and classification system for medical errors (HFACS-MES)—A Delphi study and causality analysis. PLoS One. 2024;**19**(2):e0298606

[39] Carayon P, Gurses AP, Holden RJ, King B, Perry S, Waterson P, et al. Macroergonomics in healthcare: Past, present and future of the SEIPS (systems engineering initiative for patient safety) approach. In: Proceedings of the Human Factors and Ergonomics Society Annual Meeting, Sep 2014. Vol. 58, No. 1. Los Angeles, CA: Sage Publications; 2014. pp. 1541-1545

[40] Holden RJ, Carayon P, Gurses AP, Hoonakker P, Hundt AS, Ozok AA, et al. SEIPS 2.0: A human factors framework for studying and improving the work of healthcare professionals and patients. Ergonomics. 2013;**56**(11):1669-1686

[41] Steele ML, Talley B, Frith KH. Application of the SEIPS model to analyze medication safety in a crisis residential center. Archives of Psychiatric Nursing. 2018;**32**(1):7-11

[42] Frith KH. Medication errors in the intensive care unit: Literature review using the SEIPS model. AACN Advanced Critical Care. 2013;**24**(4): 389-404

[43] Carayon P, Hundt AS, Karsh BT, Gurses AP, Alvarado CJ, Smith M, et al. Work system design for patient safety: The SEIPS model. BMJ Quality & Safety. 2006;**15**(Suppl. 1):i50-ii8

[44] Gan WH, Lim JW, Koh D. Preventing intra-hospital infection and transmission of coronavirus disease 2019 in health-care workers. Safety and Health at Work. Jun 2020;**11**(2):241-243

[45] Peerally MF, Carr S, Waring J, Dixon-Woods M. The problem with root cause analysis. BMJ Quality & Safety. 2017;**26**(5):417-422

[46] Luo G. The Use of Root Cause Analysis in American Hospitals and its Application on Chinese Hospitals. Pennsylvania, United States: University of Pittsburgh; 2013

[47] Chen TC, Schein OD, Miller JW. Sentinel events, serious reportable

events, and root cause analysis. JAMA Ophthalmology. 2015;**133**(6):631-632

[48] Liepelt S, Sundal H, Kirchhoff R. Team experiences of the root cause analysis process after a sentinel event: A qualitative case study. BMC Health Services Research. 2023;**23**(1):1224

[49] Sakdiyah SH, Eltivia N, Afandi A. Root cause analysis using fishbone diagram: Company management decision making. Journal of Applied Business, Taxation and Economics Research. 2022;**1**(6):566-576

[50] Aljadani R, Yu MC, Alosaimi A, Alsulami S, Ashkan A, Basha M, et al. Improving nursing medication administration practice in inpatient units: A quality improvement project. American Journal of Nursing. 2023;**11**(1):46-53

[51] Nicolini D, Waring J, Mengis J. The challenges of undertaking root cause analysis in health care: A qualitative study. Journal of Health Services Research & Policy. 2011;**16**(Suppl. 1):34-41

[52] Classen DC, Resar R, Griffin F, Federico F, Frankel T, Kimmel N, et al. 'Global trigger tool'shows that adverse events in hospitals may be ten times greater than previously measured. Health Affairs. 2011;**30**(4):581-589

[53] Landrigan CP, Parry GJ, Bones CB, Hackbarth AD, Goldmann DA, Sharek PJ. Temporal trends in rates of patient harm resulting from medical care. New England Journal of Medicine. 2010;**363**(22):2124-2134

[54] Cheng Y-H, Hung S-H, Ko T-W, Wang P-C. Human factor consideration in routine root cause analysis. American Journal of Medical Quality. 2020;**35**(6):507

[55] Jalali M, Dehghan H, Habibi E, Khakzad N. Application of "human factor analysis and classification system"(HFACS) model to the prevention of medical errors and adverse events: A systematic review. International Journal of Preventive Medicine. 2023;**14**:127

[56] Woodier N, Whiting K, Bennett O. Investigations by acute-hospital staff: AcciMaps or HFACS. Contemporary Ergonomics & Human Factors. 2022;**4**(2):203-214

[57] Mirzaei Aliabadi M, Aghaei H, Kalatpour O, Soltanian AR, Nikravesh A. Analysis of human and organizational factors that influence mining accidents based on Bayesian network. International Journal of Occupational Safety and Ergonomics. 2020;**26**(4):670-677

[58] Joint Commission. RCA2: Improving Root Cause Analyses and Actions to Prevent Harm. Cambridge, United States: Institute for Healthcare Improvement; 2013. Available from: https://www.ihi.org/resources/tools/rca2-improving-root-cause-analyses-and-actions-prevent-harm

[59] Kellogg KM, Hettinger Z, Shah M, Wears RL, Sellers CR, Squires M, et al. Our current approach to root cause analysis: Is it contributing to our failure to improve patient safety? BMJ Quality & Safety. 2017;**26**(5):381-387

[60] Wu AW, Lipshutz AKM, Pronovost PJ. Effectiveness and efficiency of root cause analysis in medicine. Journal of the American Medical Association. 2008;**299**(6):685-687

[61] Rooney JJ, Heuvel LNV. Root cause analysis for beginners. Quality Progress. 2004;**37**(7):45-56

[62] Card AJ. The problem with '5 whys'. BMJ Quality & Safety. 2017;**26**(8):671-677

[63] Wiegmann DA, Shappell SA. A human error approach to aviation accident analysis: The human factors analysis and classification system. Collegiate Aviation Review. 2016;**34**(2):102

[64] Shappell S, Wiegmann D. A methodology for assessing safety programs targeting human error in aviation. The International Journal of Aviation Psychology. 2009;**19**(3):252-269

[65] Wiegmann DA, Wood LJ, Solomon DB, Shappell SA. Implementing a human factors approach to RCA2: Tools, processes and strategies. Journal of Healthcare Risk Management. 2021;**41**(1):31-46

[66] Wiegmann DA, Wood LJ, Cohen TN, Shappell SA. Understanding the "Swiss cheese model" and its application to patient safety. Journal of Patient Safety. 2022;**18**(2):119-123

[67] Chen J-C, Chi C-F, Li W-C, editors. The Analysis of Safety Recommendation and Human Error Prevention Strategies in Flight Operations. Midtown Manhattan, New York City: Springer; 2013

[68] Wood LJ, Wiegmann DA. Beyond the corrective action hierarchy: A systems approach to organizational change. International Journal for Quality in Health Care. 2020;**32**(7):438-444